MY LABORATORY   MY F

AUTHOR SIGNATURE FORM

Name of book	How to be a Lab Director		
Author of Book	Philip A. Dauterman, MD	AP/CP Board Certified	Since 1996
Mandatory Comment Field	In my Pathology training days, the program strongly favored Anatomic Pathology. The Clinical Pathology training was the minimum number of months to be eligible for boards, and all classroom work. There was not even a single "hands on" course that involved on-the-job training in a real life setting. After graduation, I had a great deal of classroom knowledge, but did not know how to deal with real-life situations in real labs. I learned that on the fly and on the job. America's Pathology training programs still strongly emphasize Anatomic Pathology at the expense of Clinical Pathology. To date, there has not been an educational book written about how to be a hospital Lab Director. This book is intended to fill that void.		
Optional comment field			
Owner of book		Note: if the book ownership changes, strike the former book owner's name and affiliation with a single line and write in the new book owner's name and affiliation. All changes must be signed and dated. Use of white-out is prohibited.	
Affiliation of owner of book			
Author signature	*Philip A. Dauterman, M.D.*	**First edition published March 1, 2014**	

How to be a Lab Director
by
Philip A. Dauterman, MD

Table of Contents

Chapter 1 – Intro to the Clinical Lab

Chapter 2 – Things you probably don't need to know as a Lab Director
    A. The color on the top of the drawing tubes.
    B. Diagnostic precision and accuracy
    C. Sensitivity and specificity

Chapter 3 – How to read a Levy-Jennings chart

Chapter 4 – Pick your Westgard rules carefully

Chapter 5 – Proficiency testing and corrective actions

Chapter 6 – What to do if one analyte fails 2 or more Proficiency Testing events in one year

Chapter 7 – How to put a new analyzer into service
    A. Pick which equipment you want to buy
    B. Decide to rent, buy or lease the equipment
    C. The new analyzer and the Service Rep arrive
    D. Check correlation
    E. Do calibration and check linearity
    F. Set the Analytic Measurement Range (AMR), Reference Range and Critical Values
    G. Write the procedures for the new equipment
    H. Final preparations, going live with the new analyzer and retiring the old analyzer

Chapter 8 – How to put a new test onto an existing analyzer

Chapter 9 – How to deal with analyzer breakdowns

Chapter 10 – How to read a linearity proficiency test report

Chapter 11 – How to write a policy and/or procedure

Chapter 12 – Quality Assurance, complaints, incident reports and root cause analysis

Chapter 13 – How to deal with personnel problems
    A. How to spot a potentially homicidal employee
    B. How to spot a potentially suicidal employee
    C. How to deal with 2 lab employees that do not get along
    D. How to deal with a disagreement between employees inside and outside lab
    E. How to deal with the chronically late to work employee

Chapter 14 – Physician and administrator demands on lab and physician ordering practices

Chapter 15 – Professional relations. Making sure you are not a problem employee
    A. What to wear to work
    B. Always know your relationship to your employer
    C. Avoid conflicts of interest

Chapter 16 – Lab tech hiring, orientation, competency testing, promotion, retention and discipline

Chapter 17 – Planning and deciding which tests to do in-house

Chapter 18 – Other duties delegated to the Lab Director

Chapter 19 – How to be a Lab Supervisor

Chapter 20 – Pathologist hiring, orientation, competency testing and retirement

Chapter 21 – How to go through the inspection process
    A. How to pick an inspecting agency and prepare for the inspection
    B. The day of the inspection
    C. How to fill out CMS form 2567 and write a Plan of Correction
    D. Testing your abilities to make a Plan of Correction

Chapter 22 – Regulatory scrutiny syndrome

Chapter 23 – How to avoid HIPAA pitfalls

Chapter 24 – How to interact with the legal profession

Chapter 25 – How to be a waived test Lab Director and a PPM Lab Director

Chapter 26 – How to start a new lab from nothing

Chapter 27 – Lab Director ethics

Chapter 28 – How to prevent lab mutinies

Chapter 29 – How to chair a meeting

Chapter 30 – Lab Director hiring, orientation, competency testing and retirement

Chapter 1 – Intro To the Clinical Lab

In the US almost all lab testing is governed by a Federal law called the Clinical Laboratory Improvement Act of 1988 (known in the business as "CLIA"). There are a few exceptions, such as pre-employment drug screening. However, every Lab in the US that does patient testing must follow the CLIA regulations. As a Lab Director a good part of your time will be spent ensuring that your lab complies with all CLIA regulations.

Under CLIA there are three levels of complexity for lab testing: waived, moderate and high complexity. There is a separate entity called Provider Performed Microscopy (PPM). PPM is largely limited to outpatient clinics where the providers do their own microscopic work such as wet mounts and fern tests. In the typical hospital lab this is limited to urine microscopy, KOH prep, fern tests and wet mounts. This is an insignificant part of the typical hospital lab's workload. For this reason, I will not refer to PPM in this book again, except for Chapter 25 which deals with outpatient testing.

That being said, any given lab test is assigned to one of the three levels of complexity (waived, moderate or high complexity) based on the difficulty of doing the test. Given the way the regulations are set up, the director of a lab doing moderate and/or high complexity testing is almost always a pathologist. The director of a lab doing waived testing can be a physician of any specialty.

This book is directed mainly toward pathologists serving as Lab Director of a moderate and/or high complexity testing lab. While reading this entire book, unless stated otherwise and with the exception of Chapter 25, one can assume that the information given refers to moderate and high complexity testing. Chapter 25 deals with outpatient testing.

The typical hospital lab is divided into several sections – Hematology, Blood Bank, Chemistry, Microbiology, Urinalysis, Send-out testing, and Anatomic Pathology. The Receptionist's Office will be at the front of the lab. Immediately behind the Receptionist's Office is the drawing area.

There will typically be an office area at the back of the Lab with the Lab Secretary's, Lab Director's and Lab Supervisor's Offices.

The Lab Director is the immediate supervisor to the pathologists and the Lab Supervisor. The Lab Supervisor is immediate supervisor to the section supervisors. The section supervisors are immediate supervisors to the bench level techs. The Lab Director answers to the hospital Medical Director who in turn answers to the Hospital Administrator. The typical chain of command chart is as follows:

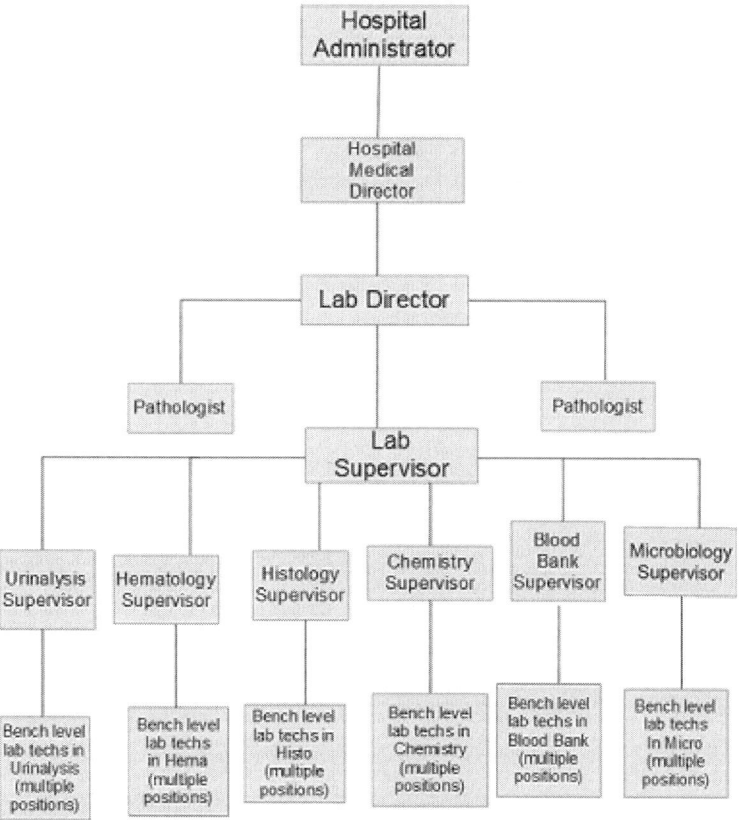

There is some variation in terminology from Lab to Lab. In some labs the position termed "Lab Supervisor" above is called "Lab Manager" or something similar.

The lab's day is divided into three shifts which typically run as follows: day shift 7AM to 3PM, evening (swing) shift 3PM to 11PM and overnight (graveyard) shift 11PM to 7AM. A lab tech working the day shift will typically work in one section only.

The term "floating" is used when a lab tech works in more than one section of lab during the same 8 hour shift. For example, if a lab tech scheduled to work in chemistry section is called upon to do Blood Bank work, the person is said to "float" to Blood Bank. The ability to work in more than one section of lab is considered a desirable quality. Not all lab techs can do this.

At some labs the evening shift and overnight shift are considered to be separate sections of lab. In this case the evening shift supervisor and overnight shift supervisor are equal in status to section supervisors. The typical small hospital lab has minimal staffing on these shifts (i.e. a "skeleton crew"). The lab techs on these shifts must work in most or all sections of lab. There is typically a pay differential for the evening and overnight shifts since these are considered undesirable shifts, and require the lab techs to "float" to most or all sections of lab.

Next I will go into filling out CMS form 209 Laboratory Personnel Report. This is required prior to all CMS inspections, and helps illustrate the relationships of the parties involved.

Here is what CMS form 209 Laboratory Personnel Report looks like:

[Form image: Department of Health and Human Services, Centers for Medicare & Medicaid Services — LABORATORY PERSONNEL REPORT (CLIA) (For moderate and high complexity testing). Form Approved OMB No. 0938-0151. Fields include: 1. Laboratory Name; 2. CLIA Identification Number; 3. Laboratory Address (Number and Street), City, State, Zip Code; 4. Instructions; 5. Telephone (Include Area Code); For Official Use Only (Not to be completed by laboratory) Qualifies According to Subpart M; Date of Survey. Positions: D-Director, CC-Clinical Consultant, TC-Technical Consultant, TS-Technical Supervisor, GS-General Supervisor, TP-Testing Personnel, CT/GS-Cytology General Supervisor, CT-Cytotechnologist. Table columns: Employee Names (Last Name, First Name, MI), Position Held (D, CC, TC, TS, GS, TP, CT/GS, CT), Shift (1, 2, 3), M or H, F or P.]

For the purposes of CMS form 209, the Lab Director is the same as the Clinical Consultant. The Lab Director provides overall supervision to the Lab. CLIA states that the Lab Director must have an MD, DO, DPM or an earned doctoral degree in science and certified by a board. The Clinical Consultant ensures the quality of reported test results and interprets test results. In all states, the interpretation of test results requires an MD, DO or possibly a DPM degree. The work of the Lab Director and Clinical Consultant typically only justifies one full time equivalent; hence one person typically fills both roles. In my experience the minimum qualification is an MD or DO degree plus Pathology board certification.

Next down the totem pole is the "Technical Consultant" in a Moderate Complexity Laboratory and the "Technical Supervisor" in a High Complexity Laboratory This is the same as the "Lab Supervisor" position in the lab chain of command diagram above. This position deals with quality control of all areas of Lab, proficiency testing, competency testing of all personnel in lab, etc.

The "General Supervisor" in a High Complexity Laboratory is more or less the same as a section supervisor in the above chain of command diagram. This position is responsible for the quality assurance of one section of Lab. This person should be able to do corrective actions and troubleshoot any problems (equipment breakdowns, controls not in, etc.) in their own section of Lab, but not necessarily for Lab as a whole.

The "testing personnel" are the people doing the day-to-day hands on work of Lab testing. Their job is to do the testing, document their work as necessary, follow the rules laid down in the procedure manual and follow instructions from their supervisors. These positions are referred to as the "bench level" lab techs in the above chain of command diagram.

Only the positions listed above go on CMS form 209. Below the bench level techs there are phlebotomists, secretaries, billing specialists, etc. Currently, I am not aware of any Lab that still has filing clerks. Currently, all hospital labs have computer systems and have done away with the filing clerk positions. None of these lower ranking positions are listed on CMS form 209

The janitorial, security, maintenance and repair positions come under the main hospital, not the Lab, such that Lab is not responsible for overseeing those positions. None of these positions go on CMS form 209 either.

After CMS form 209 is filled out you will sign it as Lab Director. Make sure to read the fine print:

READ THE FOLLOWING CAREFULLY BEFORE SIGNING

Statement or Entities Generally: Whoever, in any manner within the jurisdiction of any department or agency of the United States knowingly and willfully falsifies, conceals or covers up by any trick, scheme, or device a material fact, or makes false, fictitious or fraudulent statements or representations, or makes or uses any false writing or document knowing the same to contain any false, fictitious or fraudulent statements or entry, shall be fined not more than $10,000 or imprisoned not more than five years, or both. (U.S. Code, Title 18, Sec. 1001)

CERTIFICATION: I CERTIFY THAT ALL OF THE INDIVIDUALS LISTED ABOVE QUALIFY, TO FUNCTION IN THE POSITION INDICATED, ACCORDING TO THE PERSONNEL REGULATIONS OF 42 CFR PART 493 SUBPART M.

6. SIGNATURE OF LABORATORY DIRECTOR	7. DATE

FORM CMS-209 (09/92)   IF CONTINUATION SHEET PAGE ___ OF ___

As with most documents you will send in to the CMS, there are severe penalties for falsification. Before you sign this form, make sure the information is as accurate as possible. If you are new to that lab and have not seen the lab techs' credentials previously, double-check the credential folders for the lab techs to make sure that all the documentation is in place.

Chapter 2 – Things you don't really need to know as a Lab Director

    A. The color on the top of the drawing tubes.

While I was in medical school, The first 2 years were pure classroom work. In the third year, I did very limited drawing of patient lab specimens then went on to electives in the fourth year that involved no drawing. During Pathology residency, none of the residents did any drawing of lab specimens. From talking with other Pathologists, my education is typical of the US Pathology training system.

When I graduated from training in 1996 and took my first job, I did not know which color top tube corresponds to which lab test and vice versa. The phlebotomists and technologists considered this basic, first day on the job knowledge. The initial impression of the lab staff working under me was that my training was not very good. I had to memorize the following very quickly:

Light blue top tubes
-Contains sodium citrate which anticoagulates by forming insoluble complexes with calcium
-Used for testing coagulation (PT, PTT, INR, etc.)

Red/Black (tiger top) tubes
-No anticoagulant. Allows blood to clot. Gel acts as a barrier to separate serum and cells.

-Used primarily for chemistry panels

Red top Tubes
 -No anticoagulant. Allows blood to clot. No gel present
 -Used primarily for Blood Bank procedures and some drug testing

Green top tubes:
 -Lithium heparin (light green top) or sodium heparin (dark green top) which anticoagulates by neutralizing thromboplastin and thrombin
 -Used primarily for electrolytes and STAT chemistry panels

Lavender (purple) top tubes
 -Potassium ethylenediaminetetracacetate (EDTA) anticoagulates by binding calcium
 -Used primarily for Complete Blood Counts (CBCs)

Gray Top Tubes
 -Potassium oxalate (anticoagulates by binding calcium) and sodium fluoride (preservative)
 -Used for glucose testing and some chemistry tests

Yellow Top Tubes
 -Acid-citrate-dextrose (ACD) inactivates compliment. Citrate anticoagulates by binding calcium
 -Used for HLA typing, paternity testing and DNA studies

Orange Top Tubes
 -Contains thrombin which acts as a procoagulant.
 -Used for STAT serum chemistries

Dark blue (royal blue) top tubes
 -Sodium heparin with or without EDTA additive
 -This tube is specifically designed to be devoid of metals.
 -Used for trace element testing (zinc, copper, lead, mercury) and toxicology

Black top tubes
 -Contains buffered sodium citrate which anticoagulates by binding calcium
 -Used for Westergren sedimentation rate

Pink top tubes
 -Potassium EDTA anticoagulates by binding calcium
 -Used primarily for Blood Bank

There are a variety of special tubes on the market each with a different color on top. In general these are used for esoteric testing that you don't have to worry about.

Plasma is the acellular, liquid part of blood with the clotting factors still in it. This is what you get in a tube with anticoagulant when the anticoagulant is mixed properly with the blood. Serum is the acellular, liquid part of blood without the clotting factors. This is what you get in a tube without anticoagulant or in an improperly collected anticoagulant tube whereby the blood has clotted due to improper mixing of blood and anticoagulant.

B. Diagnostic precision and accuracy

The terms precision and accuracy appear frequently in the literature. The analogy I will give here is shooting at a target. Accuracy means having the average of your shots correspond exactly to the center of the target. Precision is how tightly clustered your shots are relative to each other.

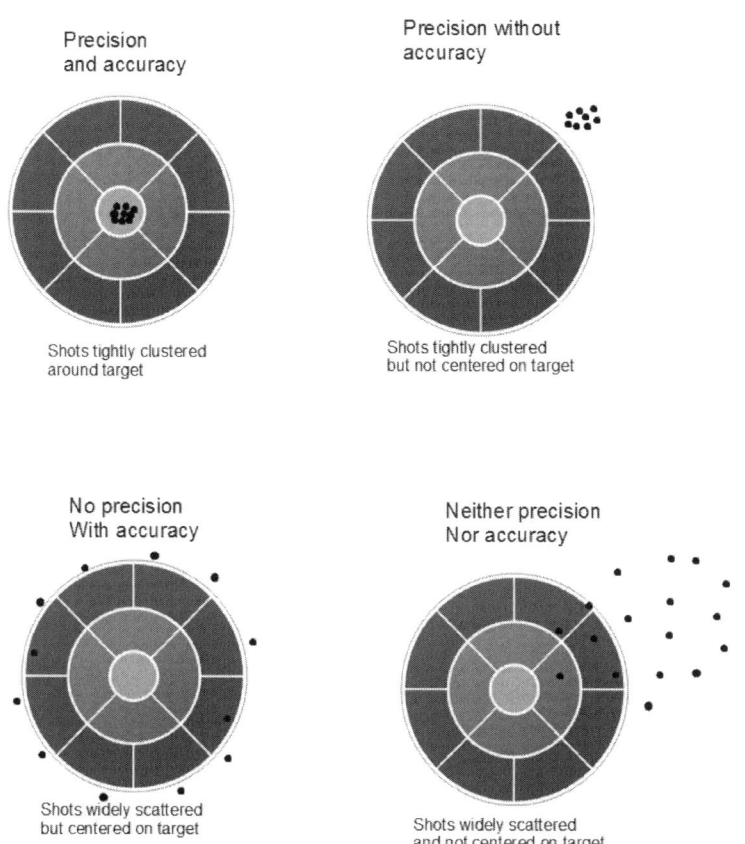

In diagnostic testing, you want to have both accuracy and precision. The main point of quality assurance is to make sure that testing is both accurate and precise.

C. Sensitivity and specificity

The terms sensitivity and specificity are heavily used in the Lab literature. When calculating sensitivity and specificity, it is assumed that the world is binary. There are only positive and negative tests, and no such thing as an equivocal or borderline test. It is assumed that the patient does or does not have a fully developed disease, and there is no such thing as a "form fruste", early stage of disease, etc.

Thus sensitivity and specificity assume a perfect binary world. In the real world, these calculations may have some value, but are overrated in my opinion.

Here's the simplest way of looking at it:

	Patient has disease	Patient without disease
Test positive	True positive	False positive
Test negative	False negative	True negative

Sensitivity = number of true positive tests divided by number of patients with disease

Specificity = number of true negative tests divided by number of patients without disease

Positive predictive value = number of true positives divided by the total number of positive tests

Negative predictive value = number of true negatives divided by the total number of negative tests

Prevalence = number of patients with disease divided by total number of patients

As an example I will use the fictitious test serum radon levels. At present there is no such test, it doesn't exist. I will use serum radon levels throughout this book as an example of a generic, garden variety test and will further assume that this nonexistent test is strongly associated with lung cancer as shown below:

	lung cancer	no lung cancer	totals
serum radon positive	99	10	109
serum radon negative	1	890	891
totals	100	900	1000

Sensitivity = 99 ÷ 100 = 99.0%

Specificity = 890 ÷ 900 = 98.9%

Positive predictive value = 99 ÷ 109 = 90.8%

Negative predictive value = 890 ÷ 891 = 99.9%

Prevalence = 100 ÷ 1000 = 10.0%

For most types of screening tests, the sensitivity and specificity depend on the cutoff used. For example, screening for prostate cancer in elderly men using PSA. If the cutoff is set very low (PSA of 2 is positive) you will have large numbers of positive tests and few of them will be true positive (prostate cancer). The sensitivity will be increased but the specificity will be reduced compared to using a middling cutoff number.

If the cutoff is set very high (PSA of 7 is positive), there will be very few positive tests, but a larger percent of those positives will be true positive (prostate cancer). The sensitivity is reduced but the specificity is increased compared to using a middling cutoff number.

In general, for population screening such as testing PSA to exclude prostate cancer, you want to have the highest sensitivity that is practicable. You don't want to miss anyone with prostate cancer, and it doesn't matter much if you do a large number of prostate biopsies. Hence, the cutoff is set relatively low for this type of testing.

Chapter 3 – How to read a Levy-Jennings chart

A Levy-Jennings chart displays data points in chronological order from left to right (x axis). Typically it represents one month's worth of controls. The y-axis is measured in standard deviations. A point one standard deviation above the mean indicates that test resulted one standard deviation above the mean, and so on.

The chart starts the month blank, as follows:

```
>3SD    _____
2-3SD   _____
1-2SD   _____
0-1SD   _____
0-1SD   _____
1-2SD   _____
2-3SD   _____
>3SD    1 2 3 4 5 6 7 8 9 10 11 12
              January
```

The chart is then filled in one day at a time. On January 7 it looks like the following:

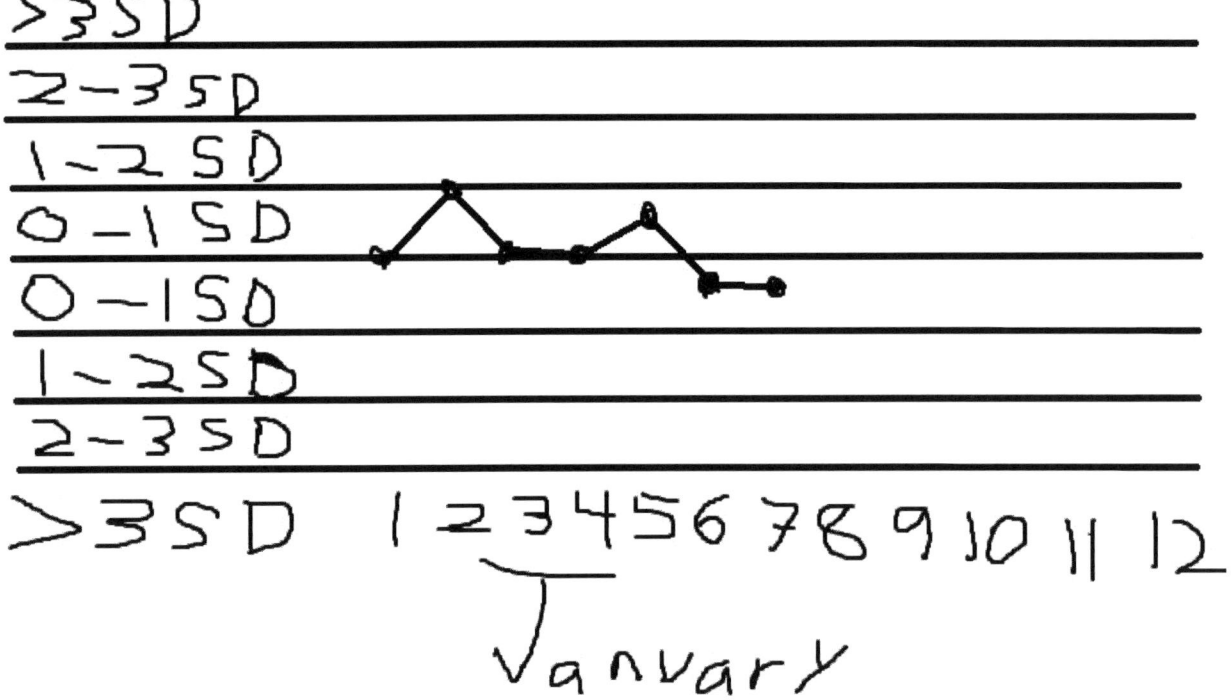

11

Eventually the chart is completely filled in

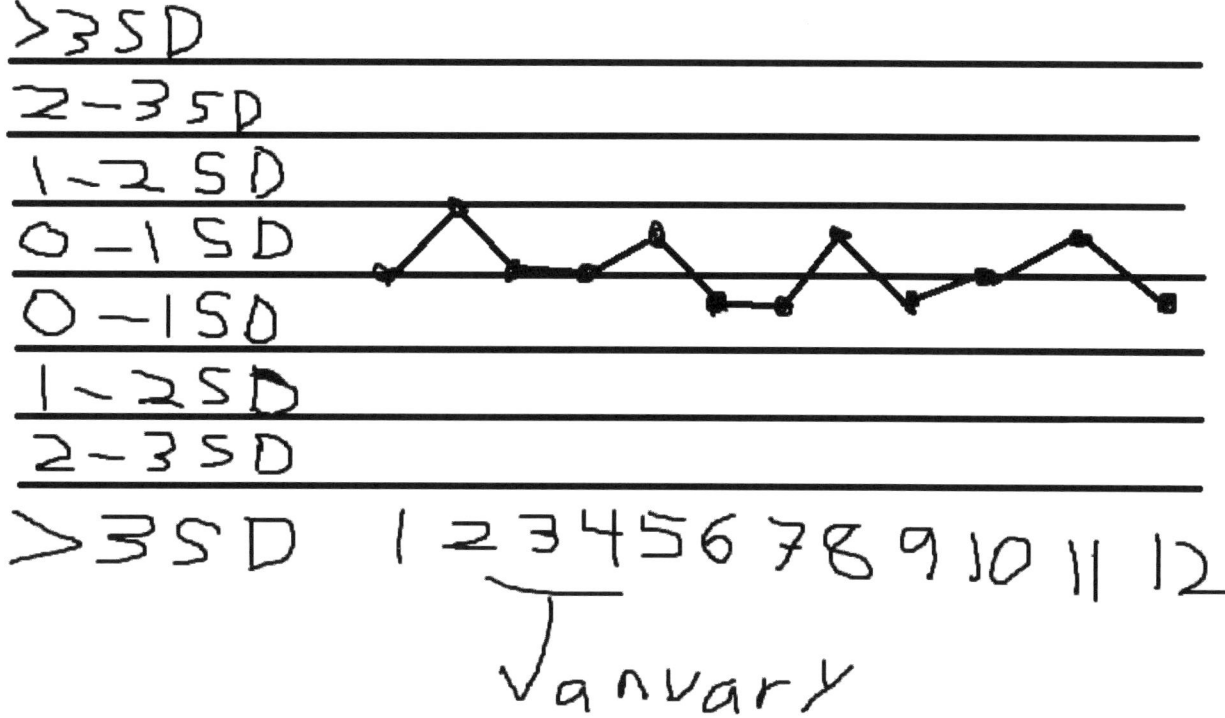

In this example, the chart only runs 12 days. That is all the time we will need to demonstrate the Westgard rules (see next chapter). In reality the typical Levy-Jennings chart runs for one or two months. The Levy-Jennings chart in the example above passes all the Westgard rules given below. The data points are clustered close to the mean, and randomly scattered above, below and on the mean.

Chapter 4 – Pick your Westgard rules carefully

In the last chapter we covered the basics of Levy-Jennings charts. In order to review these charts for quality control (QC) purposes, one must have a set of rules to determine if the chart passes or fails the rules. Multi-rule QC is called Westgard rules after the inventor. The reference is:

Westgard JO, Barry PL, Hunt MR, Groth T. A multi-rule Shewhart chart for quality control in clinical chemistry. Clin Chem 1981;27:493-501.

Extensive description of the Westgard rules can be found at the Westgard website www.westgard.com. Examples of Westgard rules are as follows:

1-3S – any one point falls outside of 3SD from the mean. In the following graph the offending data point is circled:

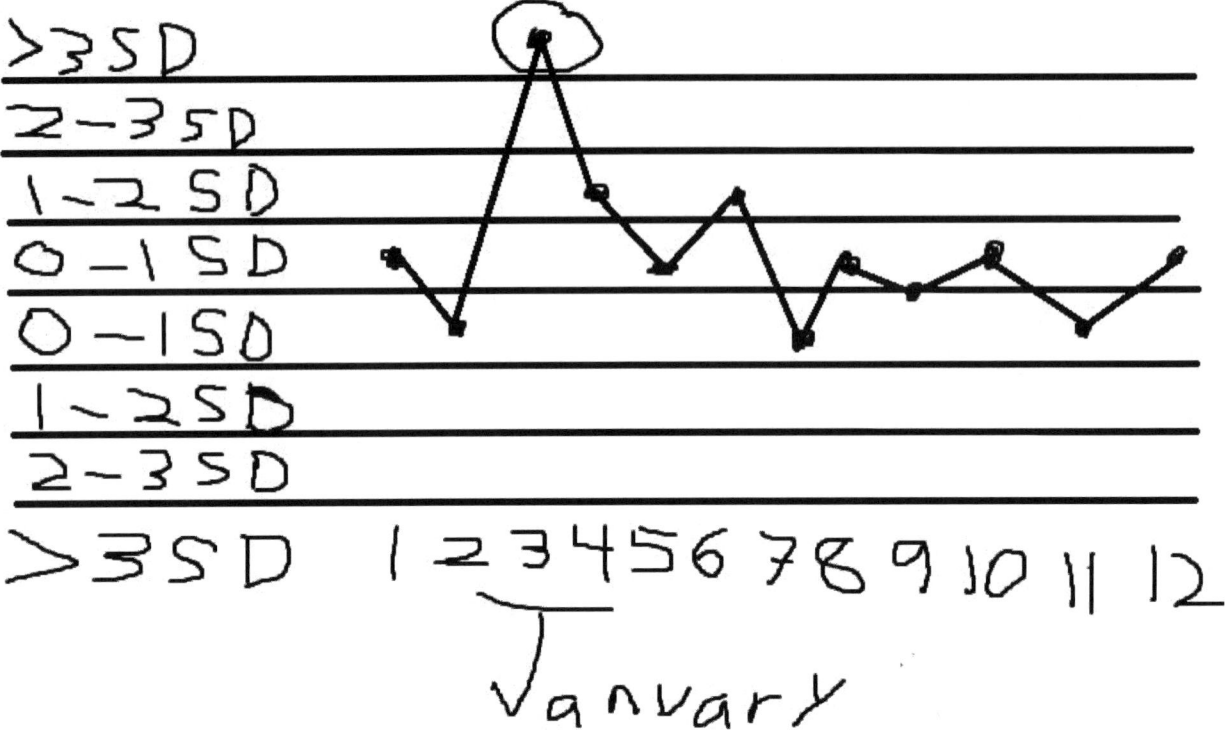

Assuming a Gaussian distribution, the probability of any given point falling more than 3SD from the mean is 0.3%. For 31 consecutive random points (a months worth of data) the chance that any one of these 31 data points will randomly fall outside 3SD is 0.3% times 31 equals 9.3%.

8x – any 8 consecutive points are on the same side of the mean. In the example below, there are 8 points above the mean, and the offending area of the graph is circled:

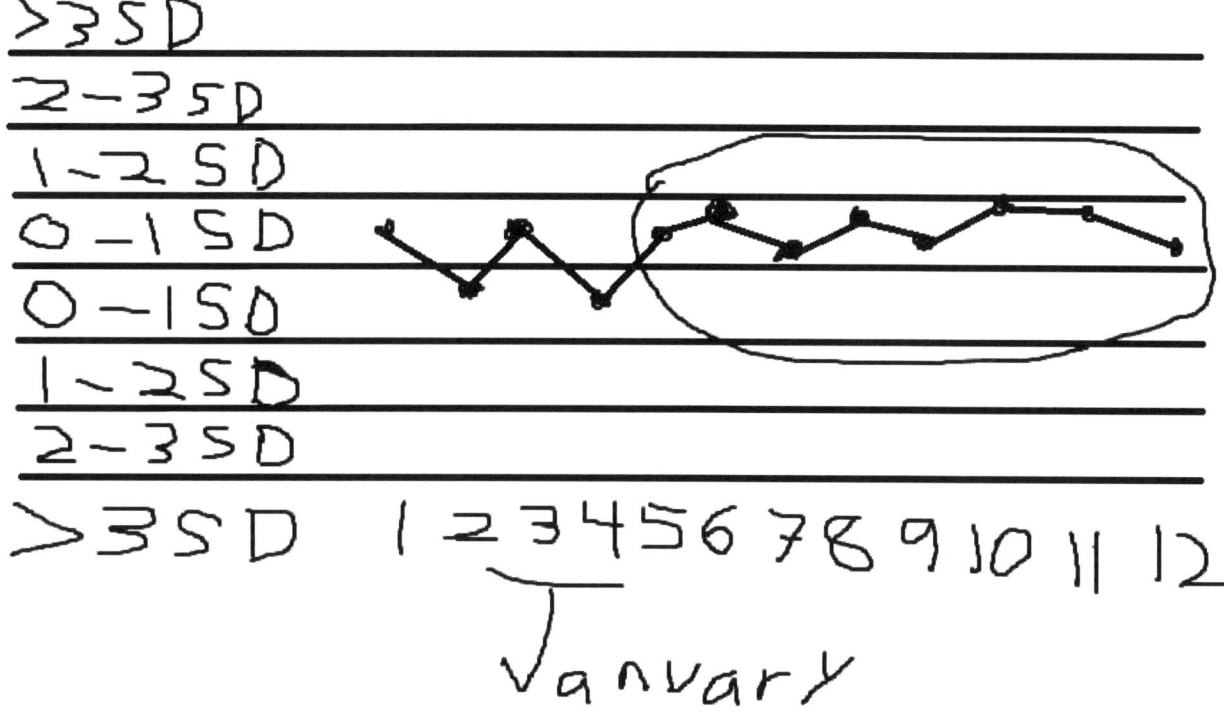

For any given number the probability of the next number being on the same side of the mean is 50%. The other 50% will be on the other side of the mean. For the purpose of this calculation we are excluding numbers on the mean. The numbers are random and discrete. This is just like a coin toss, which can be either heads or tails.

Let's say that the coin toss on day one is heads. The probability that the next seven coin tosses are heads is 0.5 x 0.5 x 0.5 x 0.5 x 0.5 x 0.5 x 0.5 = 0.78%. In the chart above the first day's data point is above the mean. The probability of the following 7 being above the mean is 1 in 2 to the seventh power, about 0.78%. Day one has a 0.78% chance of the following 7 days coming out the same. Day two also has a 0.78% chance of the following 7 days coming out the same. This continues up until day 25 at which point there are only 6 days left in the month, not enough for seven more tries. The cumulative probability over those 25 days is 0.78% times 25 equals 19.5% In the course of a 31 day month that comes out to 19.5% probability of eight consecutive data points above or below the mean by chance alone.

10x – any 10 consecutive points are on the same side of the mean. In the example below, there are 10 points above the mean, and the offending area of the graph is circled:

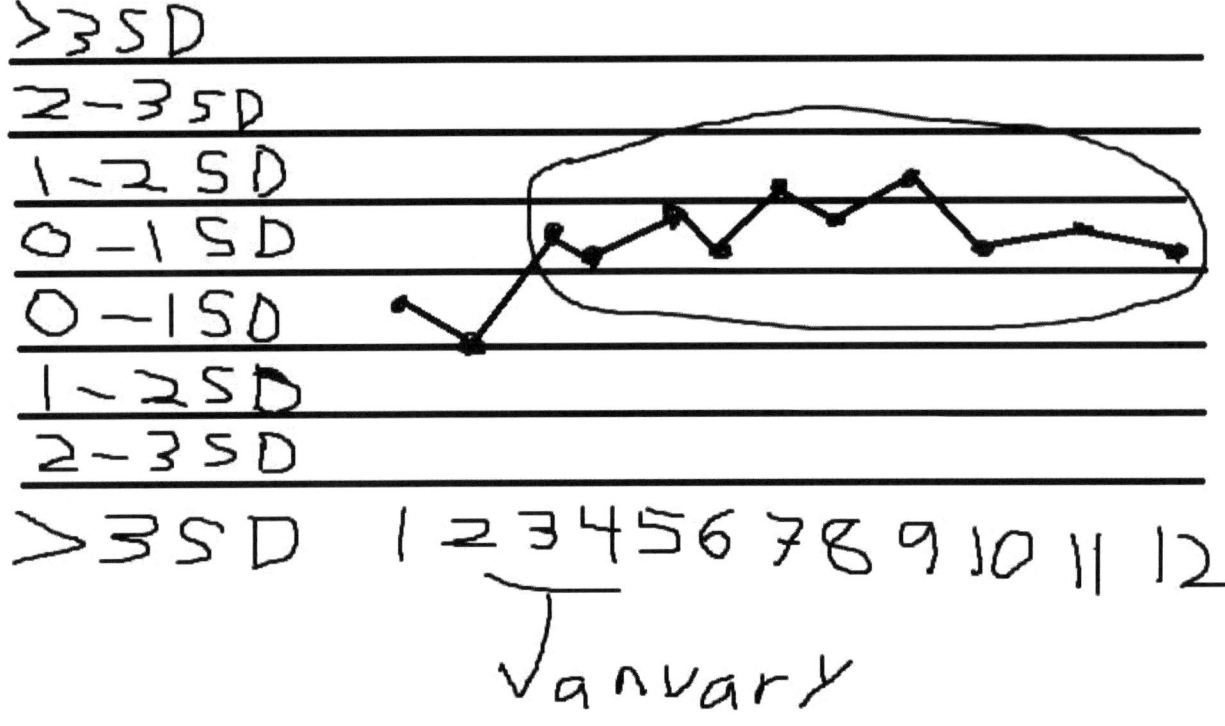

For any given number the probability of the next number being on the same side of the mean is 50%. The other 50% will be on the other side of the mean. For the purpose of this calculation we are excluding numbers on the mean. The numbers are random and discrete. This is just like a coin toss, which can be either heads or tails.

Let's say that the coin toss on day one is heads. The probability that the next nine coin tosses are heads is 0.5 x 0.5 x 0.5 x 0.5 x 0.5 x 0.5 x 0.5 x 0.5 x 0.5 = 0.19%. In the chart above the first day's data point is below the mean. The probability of the following 9 being below the mean is 1 in 2 to the ninth power, about 0.19%. Day one has a 0.19% chance of the following 9 days coming out the same. Day two also has a 0.19% chance of the following 9 days coming out the same. This continues up until day 23 at which point there are only 8 days left in the month, not enough for nine more tries. The cumulative probability over those 23 days is 0.19% times 23 equals 4.5% In the course of a 31 day month that comes out to 4.5% probability of ten consecutive data points above or below the mean by chance alone.

12x – any 12 consecutive points are on the same side of the mean. In the example below, every data point is above the mean.

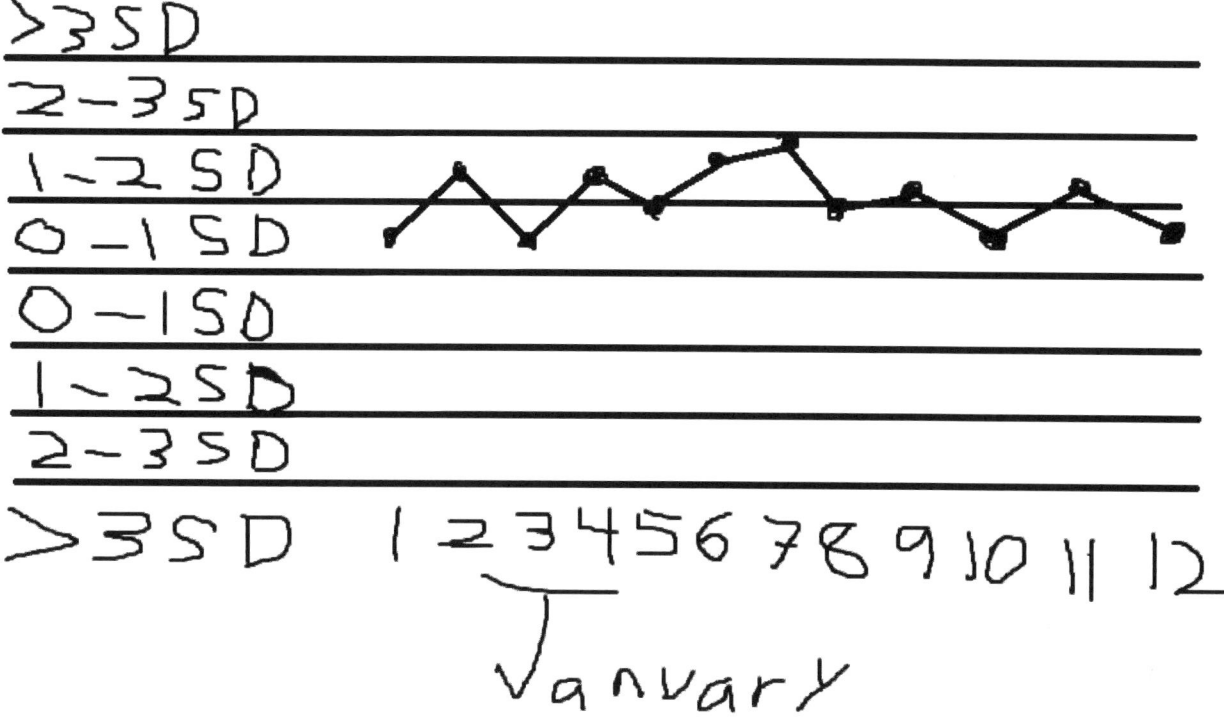

For any given number the probability of the next number being on the same side of the mean is 50%. The other 50% will be on the other side of the mean. For the purpose of this calculation we are excluding numbers on the mean. The numbers are random and discrete. This is just like a coin toss, which can be either heads or tails.

Let's say that the coin toss on day one is heads. The probability that the next eleven coin tosses are heads is 0.5 x 0.5 x 0.5 x 0.5 x 0.5 x 0.5 x 0.5 x 0.5 x 0.5 x 0.5 x 0.5 = 0.049%. In the chart above the first day's data point is above the mean. The probability of the following 11 being above the mean is 1 in 2 to the eleventh power, about 0.049%. Day one has a 0.049% chance of the following 11 days coming out the same. Day two also has a 0.049% chance of the following 11 days coming out the same. This continues up until day 21 at which point there are only 10 days left in the month, not enough for eleven more tries. The cumulative probability over those 21 days is 0.049% times 21 equals 1.1% In the course of a 31 day month that comes out to 1.1% probability of twelve consecutive data points above or below the mean by chance alone.

7t – seven data points all trending in the same direction:

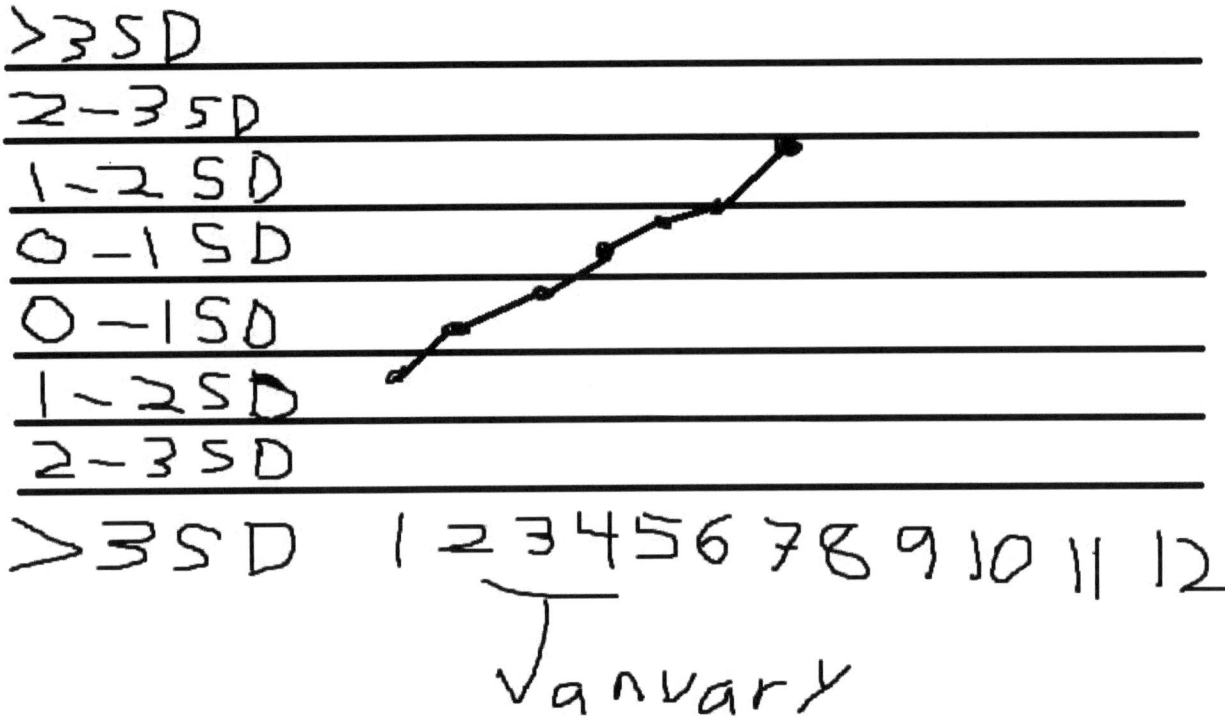

For any given number, I am making the assumption that the probability of the next number going further in the same direction is roughly 50%. This is not entirely correct since the distribution is Gaussian, but this is a rough guesstimate. Using these assumptions, this is just like a coin toss, which can be either heads or tails.

The probability that the next six coin tosses are heads is 0.5 x 0.5 x 0.5 x 0.5 x 0.5 x 0.5 = 1.5%. The probability of 6 data points trending is 1 in 2 to the sixth power, about 1.5%. Day one has a 1.5% chance of the following 6 days trending. Day two also has a 1.5% chance of the following 6 days trending. This continues up until day 26 at which point there are only 5 days left in the month, not enough for six more tries. The cumulative probability over those 26 days is 1.5% times 26 equals 40.6% In the course of a 31 day month that comes out to 40.6% probability of seven data points trending by chance alone.

10t – ten data points all trending in the same direction:

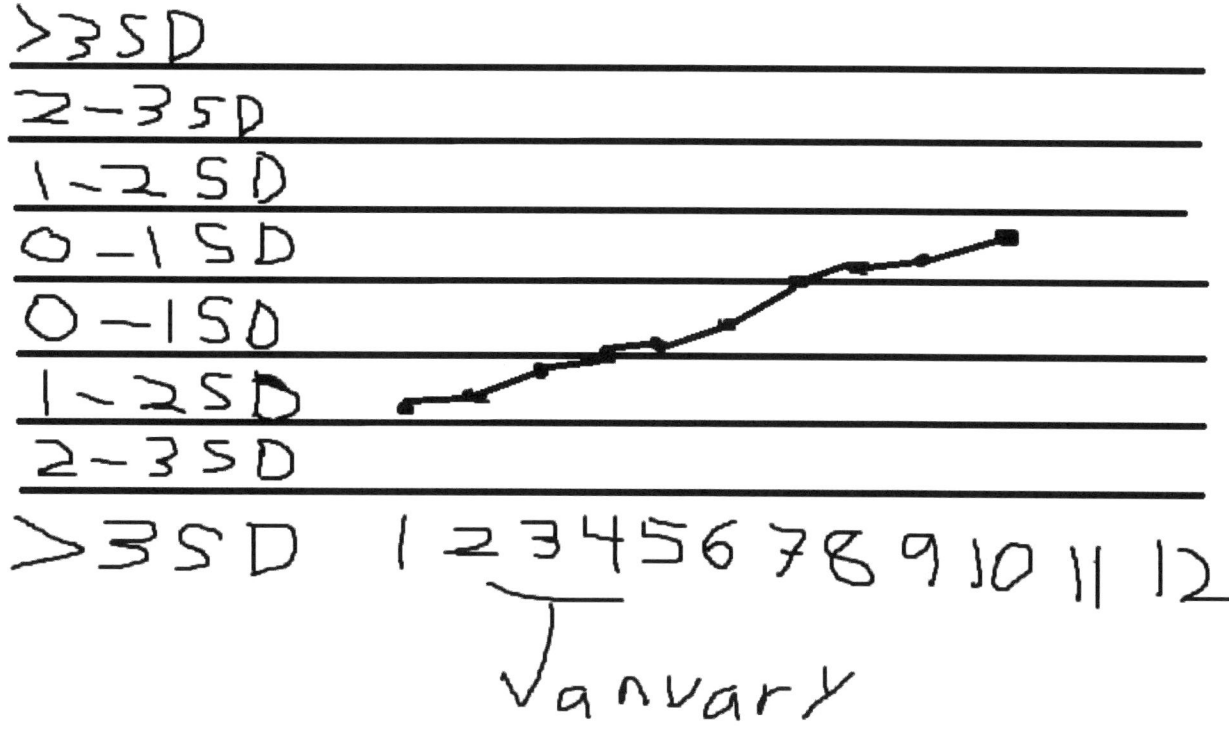

For any given number, I am making the assumption that the probability of the next number going further in the same direction is roughly 50%. This is not entirely correct since the distribution is Gaussian, but this is a rough guesstimate. Using these assumptions, this is just like a coin toss, which can be either heads or tails.

The probability that the next nine coin tosses are heads is 0.5 x 0.5 x 0.5 x 0.5 x 0.5 x 0.5 x 0.5 x 0.5 x 0.5 = 0.19%. The probability of 9 data points trending is 1 in 2 to the ninth power, about 0.19%. Day one has a 0.19% chance of the following 9 days trending. Day two also has a 0.19% chance of the following 9 days trending. This continues up until day 23 at which point there are only 8 days left in the month, not enough for nine more tries. The cumulative probability over those 23 days is 0.19% times 23 equals 4.5%. In the course of a 31 day month that comes out to 4.5% probability of ten data points trending by chance alone.

In my experience as a Lab Director, most of the Westgard rule violations I have seen on the analyzers in my lab have been "false alarms". Thus I have made a point of calculating the false positive rates for each of the tests above. In all fairness, I need to point out that the Westgard rules are very sensitive for picking up errors. In other words, if you are starting to have a problem with a test, the Westgard rules should quickly detect that there is a problem developing.

Notice that I used the monthly rate when calculating "false alarms". As a Lab Director you will review the Levy-Jennings charts, typically on a monthly basis. The tech running the equipment should be reviewing the Levy-Jennings charts daily, and if there is a problem should refer the charts to you immediately, not waiting for the next monthly cycle of chart reviews. Most modern day lab instruments can be programmed with whatever Westgard rules you want, and will flag you immediately when they begin to fail the Westgard rules they are programmed with. Keep in mind that the point of doing QC is to catch a problem as soon as possible, before it can cause any real damage.

Under CLIA, you can pick whichever Westgard rules you want. You are not obligated to pick any rule over the others. I prefer to keep it simple – three rules only: 10t, 12x and 1-3S. The theoretical probability of a false positive is 4.5% plus 1.1% plus 9.3% per month, around 14.9% per month.

Try to avoid 7t or 8x as your rules. If you pick 7t or 8x you will be forever chasing down random data points. You will spend a great deal of time and effort doing corrective actions for data points that fall by random chance in an order that fails your rules.

Theoretically, by using the 1-3S rule, about 9.3% of the time you are going to be chasing down a ghost, a point that falls outside of 3SD by random chance. In reality, what will happen is that the tech who is running QC the day of the more than 3SD outlier will re-run the control, and on the second attempt is likely to get a result within 3SD of the mean. The second attempt will be recorded as the relevant data point for the purpose of the Levy-Jennings chart.

In a perfect world, every control that falls beyond 3SD from the mean would get a corrective action. In the real world, most hospital labs are short of staff and many are very short. There isn't enough manpower to generate large numbers of corrective actions, so everybody looks the other way, and lets the tech repeat a greater than 3SD outlier once or twice.

If the repeat control results continue to fall outside 3SD of the mean, you really do have a problem. It needs a corrective action. Do not allow the tech to keep repeating the control over and over, until a number is obtained that is within 3SD. If you repeat the controls until such time as you get the desired result, it will reduce your ability to detect a real shift or trend. Set a limit that the tech can repeat an outlier only once or twice.

If the control is still outside of 3SD after the second repeat, the analyzer is assumed to be out of control. You can skip ahead to the chapter on what to do when you have failed proficiency testing, since failing QC is essentially the same thing, caught at an earlier stage. The tech cannot run tests on the analyzer and has to inform the section supervisor and/or Lab Supervisor that the analyzer is out of control. A corrective action must be completed. It must be documented that this analyzer is in control before it can be put back into service.

The same applies for all the other Westgard rules you have chosen. If your Westgard rules involve 12x or 10t and your analyzer fails 12x or 10t, the tech can repeat the offending control only twice. If the results for that control still fail any Westgard rule after the second repeat, the analyzer is taken out of commission until such time as a corrective action can be completed. The instrument can only be brought back online for testing when it is documented that it is in control.

There have been instances where the tech fails to realize that a Westgard rule has been violated, such as a quality control data point falls outside of 3SD above or below the mean. In this situation the tech will record the data point and move on as if nothing is wrong. If this happens, and you catch it at the end of the month reviewing the Levy-Jennings charts, you need to make a corrective action. If you miss this as well, and the inspector catches it, you will get a citation on the inspection. No matter how this mistake is caught, it needs a corrective action. See the subsequent chapter on proficiency testing and corrective actions.

Here is a Westgard rule **test**. Look at the following and determine if it passes Westgard rules:

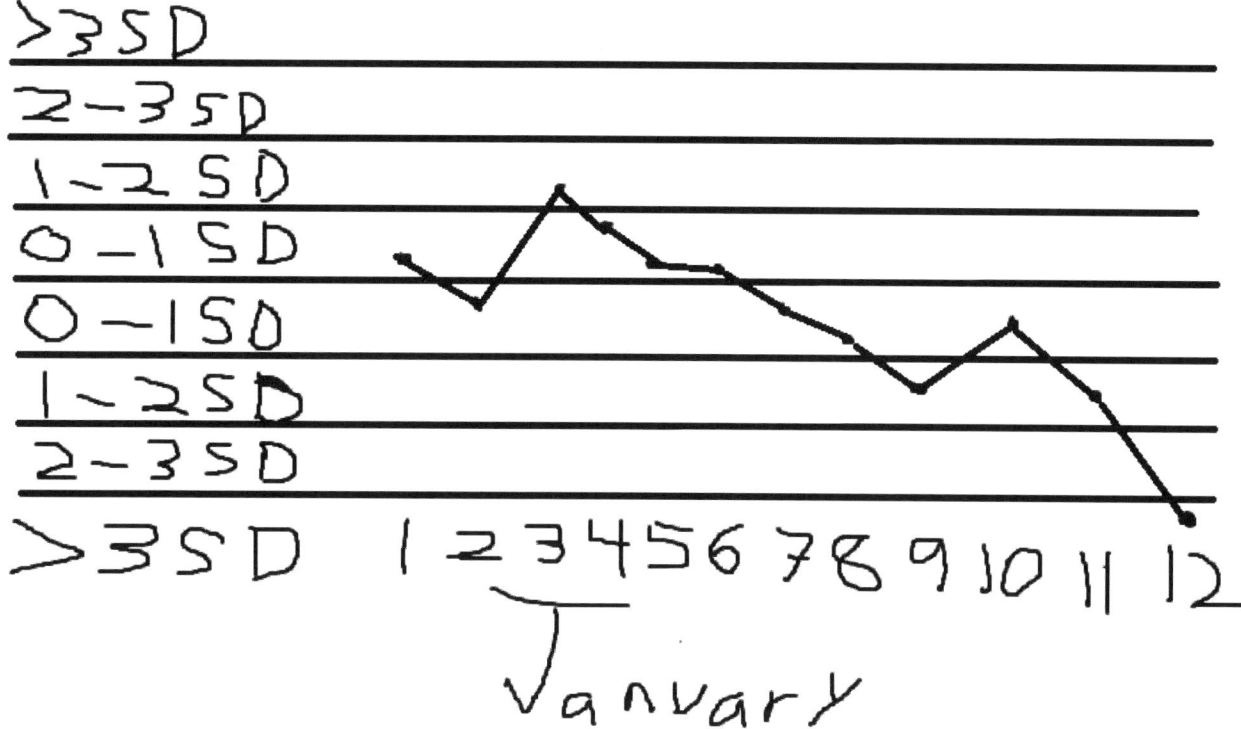

I'll give you some help on this. When looking at charts, there is a tendency to look at the middle of the chart, and miss things happening at one end or the other. This happens not only with Levy-Jennings charts, but with everything that people look at. If you take a dollar bill out of your pocket, the first thing you are going to look at is the picture of President Washington, not the numbers in the corners. You recognize this piece of paper as a dollar bill more by the picture in the middle than the numbers in the corners.

My advice: when looking at a Levy-Jennings chart, you have to look at the whole chart. Start at the left end and work your way right. Do this for each rule. Start with 1-3S. Look at every data point one at a time. Does the first data point fall outside of 3SD from the mean? Look at the second data point. Does the second data point fall outside of 3SD from the mean? Continue until you get to the last data point.

Then go from left to right on the same chart using your next Westgard rule, 7t. Look at the first data point. Do the next six points all trend in the same direction? Look at the second data point. Do the next six data points trend in the same direction? Continue until you get to the last data point.

Do this for every rule that you are using. If the chart has not failed any rules it is a passing Levy-Jennings chart. Most modern day lab analyzers can be programmed with whatever Westgard rules you want and then will automatically tell you if you are failing those Westgard rules.

I trained many years ago at a time when most analyzers wouldn't automatically flag Westgard rule failures. At that time, the evaluation of the Levy-Jennings charts were done by looking at them. The first few times you do this, it is tedious work. As you become more proficient, you will be able to do this quickly and accurately.

ANSWER: It fails both 7t and 1-3S

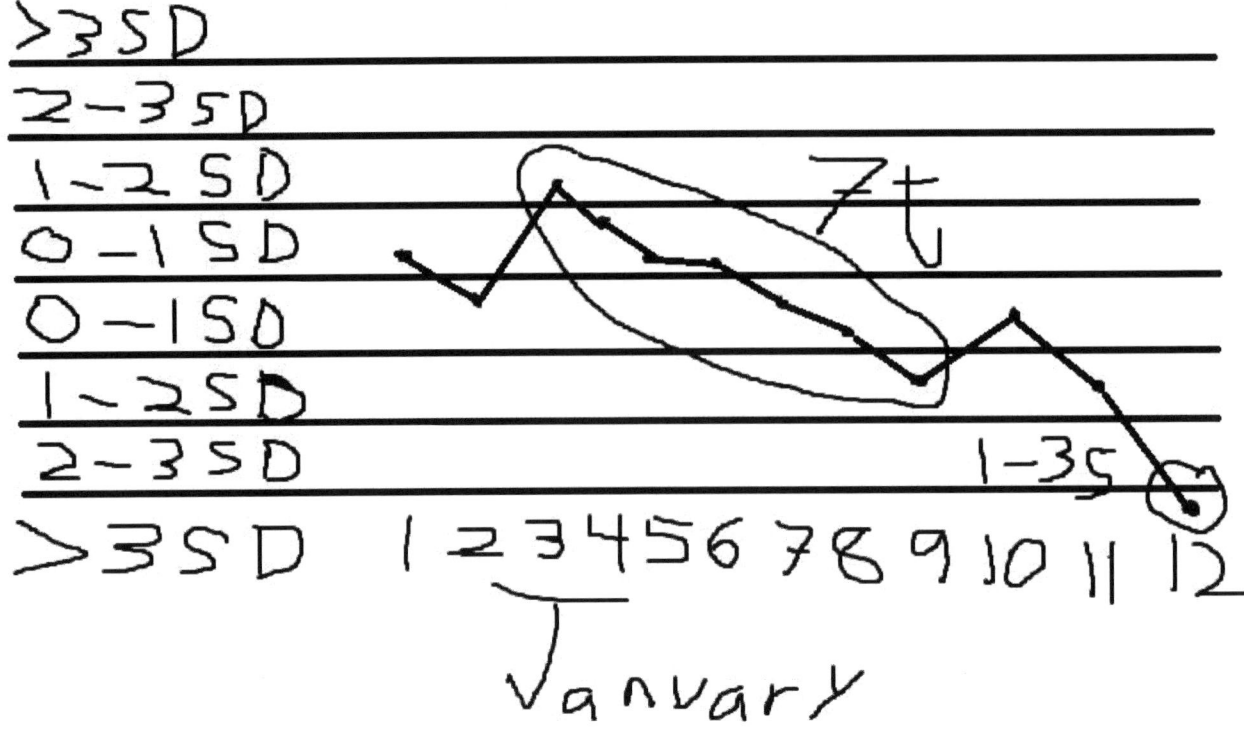

There are a number of take-home points in this graph. The first point is that the chart fails two rules at the same time. This is typical of a test that is having problems, it will fail multiple rules not just one. The analyte is having a downward trend, which results in one outlier more than 3SD below the mean. The outlier is the last data point on the chart as would be expected for a trend.

The second take-home point is to always look at the chart from end to end. If you had looked at the middle of the chart only, you would have missed the outlier more than 3SD below the mean because it is at the back end of the chart.

Chapter 5 – Proficiency testing and corrective actions

CLIA requires proficiency testing (PT) for a subset of moderate and high complexity testing analytes. Waived testing is exempted from proficiency testing. CAP requires PT for all tests in your lab. This is why I strongly prefer CMS inspection over CAP inspection, not that the inspection is easier to pass, but in between the inspections you will be doing a whole lot less work.

Proficiency testing must be done 3 times per year. CLIA requires that the PT specimens must come from a CMS approved PT provider. CLIA mandates that the testing for PT specimens must be done the same way and by the same personnel as the patient testing. The way most people interpret this is that if you have multiple techs testing the PT analyte you can pick whichever tech you want from the list of techs testing that analyte. You cannot pick a tech that does not ordinarily test that analyte. If you are testing by multiple methodologies you have to test the PT specimen by the "primary system" meaning the methodology most commonly used for patient testing.

The big sin to avoid is referral of PT specimens to an outside reference lab, or asking another lab what their results were, until such time as you have returned your results to the PT provider. If you get caught referring PT specimens your lab will be in deep trouble. The same goes for testing a PT specimen internally by multiple methodologies or multiple times. You are only allowed to do the PT testing one time by one methodology before reporting the PT results. If you break these rules, it will be considered "cheating" on your PT and your lab will be in deep trouble.

At each proficiency testing event there are typically 5 specimens sent. Many of the specimens will be lyophylized (freeze dried) and have to be reconstituted. This step is not done with routine patient testing, and this step is where the most problems arise (incorrect amount of diluent and/or wrong diluent used to reconstitute the PT sample). PT specimens tend to decay in transit, which is a bigger problem the farther away you are from the PT manufacturer.

The results then have to be transcribed onto a form, or typed into a computer to report the results back to the PT provider. This transcription step is not done with routine patient testing, and is another big source of error, in this case clerical error in data entry.

Passing is 80% for all parts of Lab except Blood Bank. Passing is 100% for Blood Bank. There are typically 5 specimens sent such that in order to pass, the Blood Bank has to get 5 out of 5 right and the other parts of Lab have to get 4 out of 5 right. Only one PT failure is allowed per year for each test. If you fail PT twice in a year for any given analyte, in theory you have to stop testing in-house for that analyte and start sending the testing out.

Each PT event will have a due date. Be very careful to return results by the due date. If you are one day late this counts as a PT failure. In my experience, this is one of the most common causes of PT failure. It is not uncommon to have one tech or even a few techs procrastinate with the PT specimens. The PT specimens can be seen as less important than the routine patient testing, and tend to be left for last, or not tested at all. In most labs it is the Lab Supervisor's responsibility to ensure that all steps in the PT process are completed in a timely manner.

Some of the proficiency testing results will come back as "educational challenge" or "no consensus". In this case, you have to compare your response to the majority response. The accompanying booklet will contain the majority responses. Write the majority response on the PT results printout. If your lab gave the majority response, document this as a handwritten note on the proficiency testing results form. All CMS inspectors like to see these types of handwritten notes, it indicates that you are paying attention to your PT. Some inspectors consider these notes to be mandatory. If you were in the minority on an "educational challenge" or "no consensus" specimen, you should make a corrective action as outlined below for a failed PT.

You are required to make a corrective action for each instance your results for an analyte are outside the expected range. For the remainder of this chapter I will refer to this situation as "failed PT". In reality, if you get 4 out of 5 right on a chemistry analyte, your overall performance is successful, but you still have to make a corrective action for the one erroneous result out of five. In effect that one erroneous result is treated as a failure even though your overall result (4 out of 5 correct) is successful.

Here is an example of a PT event where one of five failed, but the overall is passing:

T3 Uptake	CHM-11	46.00	44.376	2.130	165	+0.8	37.98	50.77	Acceptable	
	CHM-12	50.00	45.262	2.088	166	+2.3	38.99	51.53	Acceptable	C-C 2013
Percent uptake (%)	CHM-13	49.00	46.954	2.420	167	+0.8	39.69	54.22	Acceptable	C-B 2013
	CHM-14	49.00	45.226	2.010	167	+1.9	39.19	51.26	Acceptable	C-A 2013
	CHM-15	61.00	44.753	2.101	167	+7.7	38.45	51.06	Unacceptable	

x: Result is outside the acceptable limits

The lab management's response to having a failed PT varies from lab to lab. In some Labs, the failed PTs occur relatively commonly, and everybody knows how to handle them. You make the corrective action and you move on.

In one Lab I worked at, failed PT was essentially unheard of. In the year I was there, it happened one time. The Lab Director called in the Lab Supervisor, the section supervisor and the tech who did the testing into one room for a very nervous finger pointing session as to how this happened.

The corrective action is typically delegated to the section supervisor of the area where the failure occurred. Most laboratories have a corrective action form that is used in this situation. The form is filled out and signed by the section supervisor, advanced to the Lab Supervisor to review and sign, and then advanced to the Lab Director to sign off on. The corrective action form on the next page corresponds to the failed PT event given above.

My advice to the tech handed this task is that if you fail PT, take a deep breath and try to stay calm. Stay focused on filling out the corrective action form, as it will guide you in what to look for and what could have gone wrong in the PT testing.

MY LABORATORY -- PROFICIENCY TESTING CORRECTIVE ACTION/INVESTIGATION

Name of Survey	Chemistry 3rd event 2013			Date Originally Tested	10/12/13
Lab Section	Chemistry			Reconst. By	N/A
Analyte	T3 Uptake			Date Review Initiated	12/10/13
Specimen No.	CHM-15			Repeated Result	Repeated X1
Intended Result	38.4-51.0			Review Performed By	P. Dauterman, MD
Reported Result	61.00			Init / Date Completed	12/12/13
Analyte Grading	Unaccep				

SAMPLE	YES	NO	N/A	COMMENTS
Reconstituted Correctly			X	
Correct Sample Tested	X			
Correct Results Reported	X			
Correct Dilution Calc.			X	
Other				CHM-15 repeat test result 45

PROCEDURE/INSTR.				
Specify Instr				Siemens Dimension
Report Correct Meth/Instr				
P.M. Current	X			
Calibrations Done When				Most recent prior calibration 8/19/13
Calibration Since PT				Subsequent calibration 10/16/13
Reagent Problems		X		
Procedure Verified			X	
Problems on Run		X		

QUALITY CONTROL				
Within Limits		X		
Shifts Noted		X		
Trends Noted		X		
Other				

WORKSHEET				
Any Problems with PT Tests				
Any Patients Repeated				
Trend with Patients				
Other				

PREVIOUS PT FAILURE				
		X		

Final Conclusion of Above Investigation: There was no problem with controls, linearity, etc. for this analyte. The repeat test was within the expected range for this proficiency testing event. The original unacceptably high result is an unexplainable, random error.

Corrective Action to Prevent Re-Occurrence:

Evidence of Successful Corrective Action:

Reviewed By: Signature   Date   Comments

Lab Manager/Lab Director

Assuming a Gaussian distribution, the probability of a test result falling more than 3SD from the mean is 0.3%. Most analytes do not have a perfectly Gaussian distribution, but for the most part it is still assumed that 0.3% of results will fall more than 3SD from the mean by random chance alone. A proficiency testing event involves testing 5 tubes of blood for maybe 30 to 50 analytes each. Just by random chance, you might have one or two results outside of 3SD from the mean per PT event. This is referred to as "inexplicable, random error" in the form above.

In order to make this assumption, you have to exclude more sinister causes for failed PT. You have to review the controls, calibration, linearity, etc. In general the process for corrective action is:

1. Check the original machine tape to make sure there are no transcription errors.
2. Check for evidence of a specimen switch (low PT specimen had high results, high PT specimen had low results, etc.)
3. For PT specimens received lyophilized (freeze dried), make sure the reconstitution was done with correct diluent, correct amount of diluent, etc.
4. Rerun all specimens x 2 each if there is any remaining specimen to test. Record the rerun results on the corrective action form.
5. Document that all controls are in and were in for this analyte at the time of testing, the analyzer passed all Westgard rules for this analyte at the time of testing, testing for this analyte passed linearity, etc.
6. Document if PT specimen was received warm, delayed transit, etc.
7. Make notation that patient testing was not affected.
8. Sign the corrective action form and file it in with the PT testing. A copy goes in the folder for the Quality Assurance committee.

Most failed PT is a "false alarm" as described above. Any problem with the test should have been caught well before it resulted in failed PT. If you are having major problems with a test, the controls should be out for that test. This would be caught the next time the controls are run, typically once per day of testing or once per 8 hour shift depending on the test. In my experience it is very rare that the failed PT really does indicate there is a problem with the underlying test.

If you find that there really is a problem with the test you have to get the test back into control. You can try recalibration, ordering new controls, sending a split of your existing controls to an outside lab for testing to see if your controls have deteriorated, calling the analyzer manufacturer's headquarters, calling the Service Representative (known in the business as a "Service Rep") for the analyzer and ask for maintenance on the instrument and for the Service Rep to help with getting the instrument back in control, etc.

Once you get the test back in control, retest any remaining patient specimens from the time the test was out of control. If you have to turn out corrected reports for those tests, the providers who submitted the test requests must be notified of the corrected results.

You will not be very popular with any providers receiving corrected results. Even if it is a relatively minor change, for example correcting a serum sodium level from 140 to 142, it will cause your providers to distrust you, distrust your lab, and distrust your lab results. Thus, it is imperative to make sure that all tests are in control on all days of testing, so that you don't ever find yourself in the position of turning out large numbers of corrected results. It should be made very clear to all lab techs that they are not to release test results unless their daily controls are in.

You need to document that there was no patient harm from the testing that was out of control. If there was any patient harm you have to mitigate it to the extent possible. You will also need to put in place measures to prevent the same problem from recurring, and a way of monitoring this potential problem to ensure the problem does not recur. After you are done, sign the corrective action form and file it in with the PT testing. A copy goes in the folder for the Quality Assurance committee.

Chapter 6 – What to do if one analyte fails 2 or more Proficiency Testing events in one year

Per CLIA, the Clinical Laboratory Improvement Act of 1988, a lab is required to pass 2 out of 3 proficiency testing events per year. I will use as an example a test that doesn't exist – serum radon levels. Let's say that you had a transcription error earlier in the year, you switched the transcription on the high and low PT specimens, and failed your first event of the year. You passed the second proficiency test event of the year. Then on the third proficiency testing event, you incorrectly reconstituted the specimen, and failed on all 5 PT specimens for this serum radon level PT event.

Right now the last three proficiency tests in chronological order are FAIL-PASS-FAIL. The easiest thing to do at this point is to discontinue in-house testing for serum radon levels and send the test out. In some circumstances and for some analytes, the test is life or death, and you can't wait for send-out testing to come back.

Here is what you do for analytes that can't be sent out:
1. Do one more proficiency test. Order a new proficiency test from any vendor that is willing to send it immediately. Have it sent as soon as possible.
2. Do everything you can to pass the new PT test. Assign the best tech to do the testing, have a second person double-check the reconstitution of the PT specimen, double-check the transcription, etc.
3. If you pass the new PT event you will then be PASS-FAIL-PASS for the 3 most recent PT events. Only the three most recent proficiency testing events count. The first failed PT will be "pushed off the back" of the list of your 3 most recent PT events.
4. For PT purposes, you are allowed to define the year as starting on any day you want. Define the start of the PT testing year as starting somewhere in the time interval between the two failures. Thus, the two failures fall in different PT testing years.

In my 23 years in Pathology and Lab Medicine I have had two instances of an analyte in the FAIL-PASS-FAIL situation. In both instances the above steps were taken. The Lab passed the additional proficiency testing event. The CMS inspectors were satisfied with the results, or at least gave us a pass at the subsequent CMS inspection. The CMS inspectors have the ability to give citations and/or sanctions (fines) and they do not automatically pass everything.

If in step 3 above you fail the PT for that analyte you will be in a situation where the last three PT events are FAIL-FAIL-PASS. At this stage of the game, there are still a few desperate last-ditch maneuvers you could try:

1. Run 2 more PT events. Both have to pass. When the first passes, the most recent three PT events are PASS-FAIL-FAIL. After the second PT event passes, the most recent three PT

events are PASS-PASS-FAIL. You have succeeded in "pushing off the back" one of the two failing PT.
2. Put a new piece of equipment into place that employs different methodology to test the same analyte
3. Start a new lab on paper with a new CLIA number. Put this one analyte only onto the new lab's CLIA number. The new lab starts with a clean slate. Do everything that would ordinarily be done to put a new test into commission. Run three PT for the analyte.

In my 23 years in Pathology and Lab Medicine I have only once headed a Lab that had an analyte in the FAIL-FAIL-PASS situation. In August, 2013 I was hired to "turnaround" a Lab with problems. When I started work there I found that one of the problems was the sodium test results were coming out too low. The lab failed two out of the last three PT for sodium. This is an essential analyte and send-out is not an option. Here is the actual proficiency testing performance summary showing that the sodium has failed two out of the last three proficiency testing events.

CMS Peformance Summary for Analytes Regulated Under the Clinical Laboratory Improvement Amendments of 1988

CLIA ID #: ▮▮▮▮▮▮▮▮   Subspecialty: Routine Chemistry

Regulated Analyte	Proficiency Event 1			Proficiency Event 2			Proficiency Event 3			Current Event Performance Interpretation	Cumulative CLIA '88 Performance Interpretation
	Test Event	Score	%	Test Event	Score	%	Test Event	Score	%		
ALT	C-A	5/5	100	C-B	5/5	100	C-C	5/5	100	Satisfactory	Successful
Albumin	C-A	5/5	100	C-B	5/5	100	C-C	5/5	100	Satisfactory	Successful
Alkaline Phosphatase	C-A	5/5	100	C-B	5/5	100	C-C	5/5	100	Satisfactory	Successful
Amylase	C-A	5/5	100	C-B	5/5	100	C-C	5/5	100	Satisfactory	Successful
AST	C-A	5/5	100	C-B	5/5	100	C-C	5/5	100	Satisfactory	Successful
Bilirubin, Total	C-A	5/5	100	C-B	5/5	100	C-C	5/5	100	Satisfactory	Successful
Calcium, Total	C-A	5/5	100	C-B	5/5	100	C-C	5/5	100	Satisfactory	Successful
Chloride	C-A	5/5	100	C-B	5/5	100	C-C	5/5	100	Satisfactory	Successful
Cholesterol, Total	C-A	5/5	100	C-B	5/5	100	C-C	5/5	100	Satisfactory	Successful
Cholesterol, HDL	C-A	5/5	100	C-B	5/5	100	C-C	5/5	100	Satisfactory	Successful
Creatine Kinase	C-A	5/5	100	C-B	5/5	100	C-C	5/5	100	Satisfactory	Successful
Creatinine	C-A	5/5	100	C-B	5/5	100	C-C	5/5	100	Satisfactory	Successful
Glucose	C-A	5/5	100	C-B	5/5	100	C-C	5/5	100	Satisfactory	Successful
Iron, Total	C-A	5/5	100	C-B	5/5	100	C-C	5/5	100	Satisfactory	Successful
LD	C-A	5/5	100	C-B	5/5	100	C-C	5/5	100	Satisfactory	Successful
Magnesium	C-A	5/5	100	C-B	5/5	100	C-C	5/5	100	Satisfactory	Successful
Potassium	C-A	5/5	100	C-B	5/5	100	C-C	5/5	100	Satisfactory	Successful
Sodium	C-A	3/5	60	C-B	1/5	20	C-C	5/5	100	Satisfactory	Unsuccessful <3>

The Lab took option #2 from the list of possible remediations given above, putting a new chemistry instrument into service that replaced an excessively old, worn out piece of equipment. At the subsequent CMS inspection in December, 2013, the CMS inspector gave the lab a pass without any sanctions (fines), and no citations directly related to the sodium testing, new chemistry equipment, etc.

I have never had an analyte in the situation whereby the last three PT events are FAIL-FAIL-FAIL. It is unlikely that any Lab could get itself into this situation, since the analyte would be sent out after the second failed PT and/or the problem would be remediated before it came to this. My guess as to what would happen is if the analyte is truly essential to the lab you will be repeatedly called into the hospital Medical Director's Office and Hospital Administrator's Office with them expressing much displeasure with the unfolding events. Best to dust off your resume, you are in deep trouble.

My advice is that if you ever found yourself in the situation where the last three PT events are FAIL-FAIL-FAIL you would try the remediation steps given above over and over until you are successful, or until the CMS mandates that you have to stop testing for that analyte, whichever comes first. I would then try switching the testing to a waived test if possible. Put the waived test on a separate CMS certificate (i.e. a Certificate of Waiver). In theory, the CMS cannot routinely inspect a waived testing lab and can only inspect when there has been a complaint against that lab. If that doesn't work you would then be sending out an essential analyte, but you would have no other choice, you have run out of options.

Chapter 7 – How to put a new analyzer into service

A. Pick which equipment you want to buy

Lab equipment has a usable life span and depreciates over that life span. Lab equipment wears out and needs to be replaced at regular intervals. The usable life span of a lab testing instrument is around 5 to 10 years depending on the equipment.

As the equipment gets older, it will have more breakdowns. At some point it will be more expensive to continue repairing the old equipment than to buy new equipment. This is the typical point at which the decision to purchase is made.

You will need approval from the hospital's administration to buy new equipment. It tends to be very expensive, such that the decision to buy or not to buy can be very difficult. Once the old equipment has gone beyond the typical lifespan of lab testing instruments and is having frequent breakdowns, purchasing a new instrument is usually not a "hard sell" with the hospital's administration.

If the old equipment breaks down, and can't be repaired, you will be making the purchase as an emergency procurement. If you can't do basic testing like CBCs or Chem-12s and end up sending them out for testing, the medical staff will be very upset with the turnaround time. In this situation the hospital's administration will be signing all the equipment procurement paperwork you bring them and worrying about the cost later.

For most types of equipment (chemistry, hematology, etc.) there are multiple manufacturers to chose from. Typically the decision as to which one to buy from is made based on economics – pick the cheapest vendor. Sometimes the decision is made based on convenience – if every other lab in your community uses one vendor, you should as well so that you are able to share reagents with the surrounding labs.

CLIA makes the Lab Director responsible for "appropriate test method selection". In my experience the equipment is selected based on which manufacturer is the cheapest to deal with. I don't really care if the instrument is using radioimmunoassay (RIA), enzyme linked immunosorbent assay (ELISA) or other methodology. I really only care that the testing has precision and accuracy.

All clinical testing manufacturers have to get their equipment to pass FDA standards in order to sell their equipment in the US. Thus, one can assume that any equipment being sold in the US meets the minimum standards for clinical lab testing. As far as I am concerned as a Lab Director, the methodology used, RIA versus ELISA versus other methodology, doesn't really matter.

The big caveat here is to make sure that the new piece of equipment does not have special requirements that exceed the specifications of your existing facility. Is the new piece of equipment too large to fit in the existing space? Does it have requirements for a special type of water, narrow temperature and/or humidity requirements? Will it need special ducting for contaminated exhaust air? You don't want to buy a piece of equipment only to find that you have to move your whole lab into a larger space to accommodate the new equipment, ducting for the new equipment, etc.

B. Decide to rent, buy or lease the equipment

It is possible to buy, rent or lease lab equipment. This is just like any other piece of capital equipment, such as a car.

For lab equipment, lease arrangements are the most common in my experience. Leasing has many advantages over buying. Leasing has less up-front costs compared to buying. If the equipment breaks down, the leasing company has to repair it. At the end of the lease term, typically 5 years, you can trade in the old instrument for a brand new instrument while making a new lease. Alternatively, the lease can be set up so that you can buy the equipment at the end of the 5 years and obtain outright ownership of the equipment after the lease is over.

The main disadvantage to leases is that the interest rate is typically variable. If interest rates go up, you will be paying more for the lease. However, if interest rates go down, you will be paying less for the lease. In the business world uncertainty is unnerving. It is hard to budget for a lease if you don't know how much next year's payments will be.

Another disadvantage of a lease is that you are legally committed to the deal for the term of the lease, which is typically five years. It is possible for a test or technology to become obsolete in less time. If you had leased equipment to do CK-MBs at the same time your competitor down the street got troponins going on their equipment, you would have been out of luck, stuck with obsolete, unused equipment for the remainder of the lease.

Reagent rental is another option. In this option you pay per test. There is usually a minimum payment based on the minimum number of tests that will be done. This option is best for reference labs doing a large volume of testing. Even if you don't meet the minimum number of tests you will still have to pay the minimum payment, in effect paying for tests that are not done.

After making the decision to buy, rent or lease, the next step is to negotiate the price and other terms with the vendor. After reaching agreement on all terms, the hospital and vendor sign an acquisition contract. Most hospitals have a Materials Management or Procurement Office that will handle most of the purchase paperwork. After the paperwork is executed, the vendor will send the equipment. Usually the hospital pays for the transport of the equipment. The vendor should supply you with enough reagents and supplies to get you started.

C. The new analyzer and the Service Rep arrive

The new analyzer will arrive a few days to weeks after the acquisition contract is signed. In general most of the work of putting a new analyzer into service will be done by the Service Representative (known in the business as a "Service Rep"). The Service Rep is a traveling representative of the company that made the analyzer.

The Service Rep tends to be more of a hardware person than a quality assurance person. As such, the Service Rep typically has technologists available for phone consultations from the company headquarters. These techs know more about quality assurance, but they rarely leave the corporate headquarters and you will likely never meet them in person. You are allowed to call these techs directly without needing to have the Service Rep on the line.

If the analyer has quality assurance problems (fails controls) that you can't mitigate internally, call the company headquarters first. If the analyzer has an issue that is obviously a hardware problem call the Service Rep first.

Almost all analyzer acquisition contracts state that the company must approve of any and all changes to the analyzer or else these changes will void the warranty and servicing agreement. The Service Rep is your point of contact for the company that made that analyzer. As such the Service Rep has the authority to decide what changes the company will or will not allow to the analyzer.

The Service Rep will also do all the maintenancing for that analyzer, flying in a few times a year to do this work. The Service Rep can be called in on an unscheduled basis if there is a major problem with the analyzer such as the analyzer goes down and can't be brought back up again.

As soon as the analyzer arrives on site the Service Rep should fly in to do the calibration, correlation, linearity, etc. Your staff should not have to do the majority of this work.

D. Check correlation

Correlation is tested by running split samples on the old instrument and the new instrument. The lab tech takes at least 20 random patient samples, splits them and runs them all on both the old instrument and the new instrument. The results are used to calculate the correlation of the new instrument to the old instrument.

Usually the Service Rep calculates the correlation, but this calculation can also be done by the Lab Supervisor. Alternatively, the raw data can be E-mailed to the analyzer manufacturer's corporate headquarters for them to do the calculation. The results are usually expressed as correlation coefficient (R). The correlation testing is usually reviewed by the Service Rep and Lab Supervisor for their approval and then brought to the Lab Director to sign off on.

R can range from -1 (perfect negative correlation) through zero (no correlation) to +1 (perfect positive correlation). In my experience the typical R for comparing one piece of equipment to another is at least 0.98. For setting new equipment into service, most people in the profession, myself included, prefer an R of 0.95 or higher.

Here is an example of a correlation that was used to put a new piece of equipment into service:

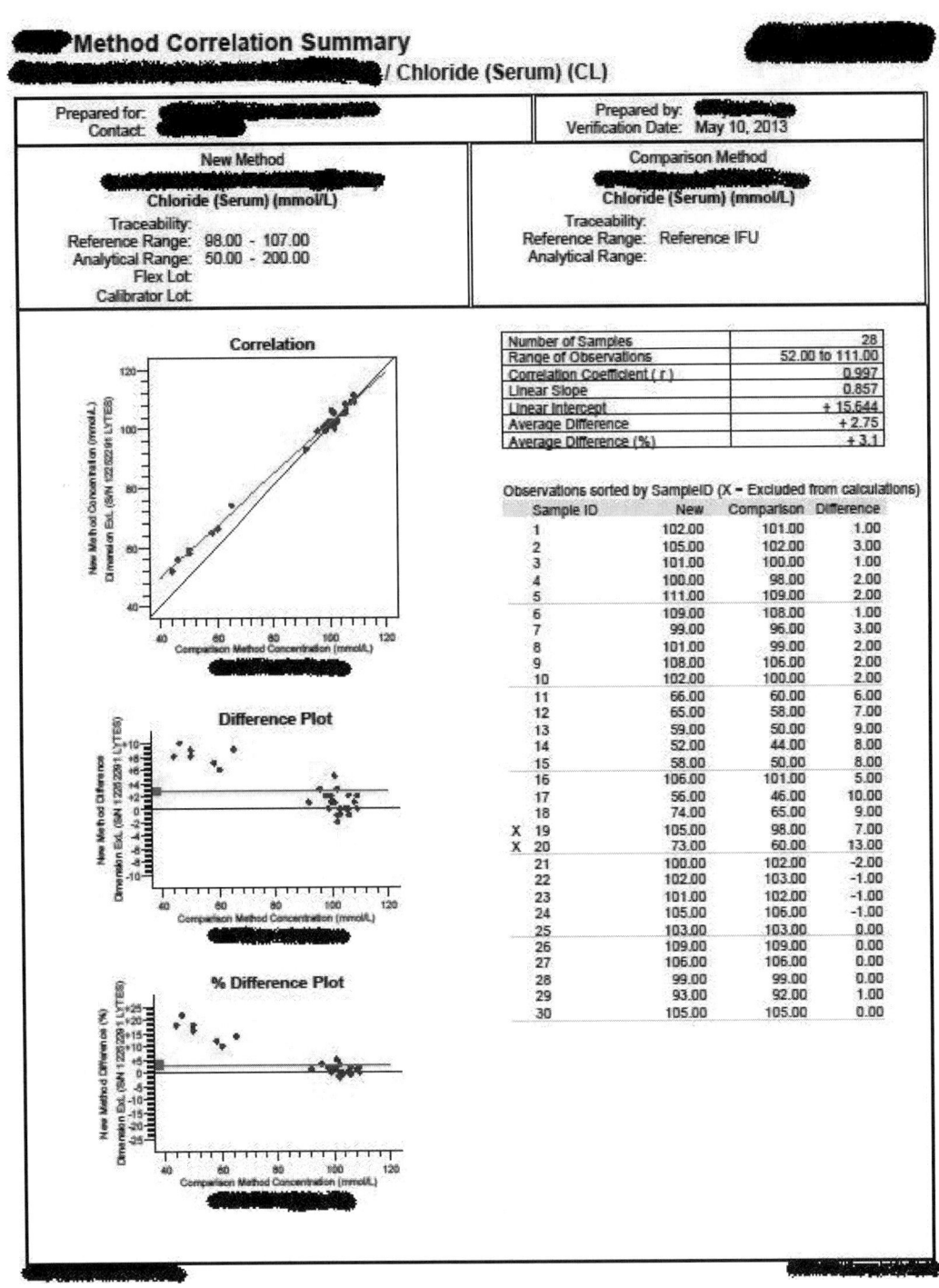

This correlation came out to 0.997 which is near perfect. Perfect positive correlation is 1.000. When you see a correlation this good you don't have any hesitation on accepting it. Just sign it and move on. If the correlation comes out to less than 0.95 that is when I start getting worried that something is wrong.

CLIA does not set a minimum for correlation. If the correlation comes out below 0.95 you can accept that if you want. If the correlation comes out below your expectation, you can improve it by running some more samples. Use a few very low (or negative) samples and a few very high samples.

The very high samples should be just below the cutoff of the Analytic Measurement Range (AMR). Do not exceed the AMR on either instrument or you will cause yourself more problems than the low correlation problem you are trying to solve.

You will find that adding in a few very low and very high samples will drive the correlation coefficient up to nearly +1, near perfect positive correlation. I have heard of some Clinical Chemistry people referring to this technique as "cheating". Keep in mind that CMS does not specifically forbid this technique. It's a free country, you can do whatever you want unless there's a law or regulation against it. There is no law or regulation to stop you from running very high and very low specimens to improve your correlation.

If your correlation is still below 0.95 after doing this, I would have serious reservations about accepting the instrument that just arrived. I would be discussing the problem with the Service Rep and telling the Service Rep there seems to be a problem with the new instrument. It looks like lack of precision on the part of the new instrument and I am thinking about asking for a replacement for the new instrument.

E. Do calibration and check linearity

A calibrator is a sample containing a known quantity of an analyte. CLIA requires a minimum of 3 calibrators – low, normal and high. Calibrators are typically purchased, usually from the manufacturer of the instrument that will be calibrated using that calibrator. When you purchase calibrators, they will come as a set of at least 3 and possibly as many as 5 of the calibrator material.

The low calibrator should test the low end of the Analytic Measurement Range (AMR). This is zero for most analytes. There should be a middle calibrator that roughly corresponds to the middle of the reference range. The high calibrator should be just below the upper end of the AMR.

The calibration is typically done by a bench level lab tech or the section supervisor of the lab section where the equipment is situated. The calibrator samples are run on the instrument. The results obtained from the testing are compared to the known/expected value of the calibrator specimens.

If the instrument gives out results within a percent or so of the expected values the lab tech accepts things as they are. If the instrument gives results that are significantly different from the expected, the tech reprograms the instrument so that it gives out the expected results.

Calibration verification refers to testing a specimen of known concentration in the same manner as a patient specimen to verify the instrument's calibration throughout the AMR. Calibration verification is required by CLIA if the test has not been recalibrated for 6 months. You will need to do this prior to setting your new piece of equipment into service.

Calibration verification is easy. All the lab tech has to do is re-run the same calibrator materials after the calibration. Since you've already calibrated the instrument to that calibrator, you're almost guaranteed to pass the calibration verification.

For some analytes, you will receive only 3 calibrators. If you are doing calibration verification and want to test the entire AMR using multiple different known amounts of analyte, you can draw an aliquot from the various calibrators, and mix them to make multiple different samples of known quantity.

For example if the low calibrator has zero of the analyte and the middle calibrator has 100, you can mix the low and middle calibrators 1:1 and assume that the resulting mixture has 50 of the analyte. If the middle calibrator has 100 of the analyte and the high calibrator has 300, you can mix the middle and high calibrators 1:1 and assume that the resulting mixture has 200 of the analyte. If the low calibrator is not zero, you can use saline as a zero calibrator, etc. You can mix saline 1:1 with any of the three controls (low, middle and high) to make a mixture of known concentration. In this manner it is possible to perform calibration verification by testing multiple points throughout the AMR.

Precision is defined as having multiple repeat results closely approximating each other. Precision is tested by making multiple repeat tests of the controls. Usually this is limited to 3 repeats of each of the controls.

Allowable imprecision under CLIA is given in a series of tables printed in the Federal Register, the reference is February 28, 1992;57(40):7002- 186. In looking over these tables, CLIA allows a huge amount of imprecision. For example for HDL cholesterol you are allowed to be up to 30% off from the target value. In my experience when repeating the HLD cholesterol middle and high controls over and over, they will not usually be off from each other by more than a percent or two. Multiple repeats of the HDL cholesterol low control (i.e. not a zero control) may be off from each other by a few percent.

Aiming to pass the CLIA criteria for precision is like trying to shoot a barn door; it is so wide you can't miss. Hence, I have never seen an analyzer fail testing for precision. The requirements for controls being within 3SD of target are much narrower than the huge variation allowed in precision. Hence, when an analyzer starts having problems it is bound to fail controls before it fails precision.

Linearity refers to the range in which the test result holds a straight line relationship to the analyte. Linearity is very similar to AMR.

Let me explain how linearity and AMR are similar. For example for HCG below 100,000 if you increase the "true" concentration of HCG by +1, the instrument will report a +1 increase in HCG. However, at the extreme upper range of an analyte the instrument may begin to give non-linear results.

Above 100,000 HCG the testing capability of the instrument may get saturated. These tests are typically enzymatic or immunoassays, and above 100,000 HCG most of the enzymes or antibodies used for testing are already saturated with HCG. In this range a +1 increase in the "true" HCG concentration may result in less than a +1 increase in the test result. If this happens, the instrument is now outside its linearity range.

The test results for these extremely high, non-linear HCG measurements tend to be unreliable. Unreliable results cannot be reported. Thus, these extremely high HCG results are outside the AMR as defined below. In other words, with increasing concentrations of analyte as soon as the linearity of the test is exceeded, the results usually becomes unreliable and can't be reported. Therefore the linear range tends to be identical to the AMR.

CLIA has no requirements for linearity but does have requirements for AMR, so I will spend more time discussing AMR than linearity. In order to set your new piece of equipment into service, you should order one linearity PT event.

When the instrument is being set into commission it is very uncommon to have problems on a linearity PT in my experience. The linearity is identical to the AMR, and the manufacturer has already set the AMR, so you should be good to go. See below. If you fail any part of the linearity PT, do corrective action as outlined above.

While the instrument is in use the linearity will be repeated every six months or year. If the instrument becomes non-linear for any analyte this could be an early warning sign that you are having problems with that particular test. The linearity tends to go out first, before the test goes out of control. See the section above on corrective actions to deal with this situation.

F. Set the Analytic Measurement Range (AMR), Reference Range and Critical Values

The Analytical Measurement Range (AMR) is the range of analyte concentration that the instrument can measure without pretreatment (i.e. dilution) of the sample. The reportable range refers to the range of test results for which the laboratory can verify the accuracy of the test

I will use again the example of HCG given above. If the test becomes non-linear above 100,000 then the AMR is set by the manufacturer as zero to 100,000. If a specimen has an HCG above 100,000, the instrument will flag the specimen as too high to test, and printout a result of ">100,000".

The lab can either report the specimen as "Greater than 100,000" to try to dilute the specimen and run it again in a diluted state. Let's say the specimen is diluted 1:1 with saline and rerun. The instrument now reports a result of 76,000. You multiply the result by the dilution factor to come out to the "true" HCG result of 152,000. This can be reported with the caveat (usually in a comment) that the test result exceeds the AMR of the instrument and the specimen had to be diluted in order to test it.

In the example of the diluted HCG specimen given above, the AMR of the instrument is 100,000 but the reportable range of the test is 200,000. CLIA requires that in order to use this expanded reportable range, the lab needs to run calibration and calibration verification for the expanded reportable range (100,001 to 200,000 HCG in this example)

In regard to setting a new piece of equipment into service, all you need to do is accept the manufacturer's AMR. I have never seen any lab determine an in-house AMR for each analyte. This would be very difficult to do, very time consuming, and would not add much value. All you have to do is accept the manufacturer's AMR and move on.

The term "reference range" refers to the range of test results that you would expect to see in a normal, healthy individual. For the most part labs simply accept the reference range of the manufacturer.

I have seen a few labs make their own reference range for a few analytes, but this is uncommon. The reference range is frequently defined as the central 95% of test results of normal, healthy individuals. To make your own reference range, you will need to draw 40 normal, healthy people and test their specimens. The 38 median results are the reference range. In other words, starting with 40 normal people's test results discard the highest and lowest outlier from the 40 normal tests. The highest and lowest of the remaining 38 represent the reference range.

There is very little variation in serum chemistries, hematology, etc. in normal, healthy people. Thus, making an in-house reference range is like re-inventing the wheel - it has been done before. You have to stick 40 normal people to get specimens just the same way that the manufacturer had done when making the manufacturer's reference range.

In my experience any reference range made in-house tends to be almost identical to the manufacturer's reference range. You are measuring the exact same thing - chemistry and hematology tests in normal, healthy people, so it is not unexpected that you get the same results.

You have just stuck 40 people to get specimens, and the whole exercise was a waste of time and effort anyhow. You are right back where you started, with essentially the same reference range. It is much easier to accept the manufacturer's reference range from the start.

The term "critical values" refers to any lab result that could be life threatening. This was formerly referred to as "panic values". Such test results must be immediately called to the ordering provider, with documentation of the call. Most labs accept the manufacturer's critical values. I have seen a few labs set their own critical values for some tests.

G. Write the procedures for the new equipment

When putting a new piece of equipment into commission the manufacturer will oftentimes supply you with procedures. These are fill in the blank forms whereby you paste the name of your hospital in the blanks, print out the procedures, and file them in a procedure manual.

If the manufacturer won't supply you with procedures, you can try the following. Numerous hospitals keep there procedure manuals online, such that it is possible for anyone anywhere to download their procedures. All you have to do is find a hospital that is using the same equipment, download their procedures, change the name to your lab's name, print out the procedures, and you've got a procedure manual.

If the above doesn't work, you will end up writing the procedure manual yourself. See the chapter below on how to write a procedure.

H. Final preparations, going live with the new analyzer and retiring the old analyzer

In most labs the Lab Supervisor is responsible for ordering all the supplies, reagents, PT specimens etc. When a new instrument comes on line, the Lab Supervisor will need to set up standing orders (orders for routine delivery) of supplies and reagents for the new instrument, and discontinue ordering of supplies and reagents for the old instrument.

The standing orders should include orders for controls. A control is a specimen with a known amount of an analyte. This is very similar to a calibrator. The difference is that calibration is done at 6 month intervals and designed to set the instruments results to match the calibrator. A control is run on each day of testing (or more often) to verify that the instrument is giving good responses. Running controls does not reset the instrument's results while running calibration does. Otherwise calibrators and controls are similar.

Controls can be either assayed or unassayed. Assayed controls are typically made by the manufacturer of the analyzer and are specific to that manufacturer's analyzer. In other words if your chemistry analyzer is made by Siemens, you can't use Abbott assayed controls on it, you can only use Siemens assayed controls on it. The assayed control has a known amount of the analyte. The mean, standard deviation and expected range are provided by the manufacturer. Assayed controls are more expensive, but they are generally worth it since the manufacturer has done extensive testing on that control before sending it to you.

Unassayed controls do not have a known amount of analyte. The mean, standard deviation and expected range are not provided by the manufacturer. This is typically limited to microbiology where a culture is either positive or negative for an organism.

Essentially all hematology and chemistry controls are assayed controls. If you used an unassayed control on hematology or chemistry analyzers, you'd have to determine the mean, standard deviation and expected range of the control on your own analyzers. You would then use that control to check if your own analyzers were in control. You would be comparing your own analyzers to your own analyzers, not the rest of the world. Thus, an unassayed control would be useless in this setting. For the remainder of this book, when referring to a "control" I will be referring to an assayed control.

All labs that I am aware of purchase their controls from a vendor, typically the manufacturer of the analyzer. It is possible to make your own controls in-house but I have never seen a lab do this. Making your own controls would be too time consuming, costly and the controls would be unassayed controls.

The test is said to be "in control" if the results of testing correspond to the expected values from the known amount of analyte in the control specimens. If not the test is said to be "out of control". In general, troubleshooting for out of control tests falls first on the bench level tech operating the instrument, next on the section supervisor and then on the Lab Supervisor. If not fixed relatively quickly, calls will be made to the analyzer manufacturer's headquarters and/or the Service Rep for the instrument.

In my experience a new piece of equipment is almost always in control. I have seen one or two instances where a new instrument came in out of control, but was easy for the tech to bring back into control. I have never seen a new piece of equipment repeatedly fail controls. If your new piece of equipment is out of control, and none of the techs can get it into control, and the Service

Rep can't get it into control, it would mean that you had just received a defective piece of equipment. Reject this instrument and tell the manufacturer to take it back and replace it with a new one.

If you are testing the same analytes on the new instrument as the old instrument you don't need to rearrange the PT ordering. You do need to inform the PT manufacturer of the change in equipment. The calibrators tend to be specific to one type of analyzer, so you may need to change the ordering of calibrators.

If there are any tests added or deleted from the test directory, the ordering of PT, calibrators, etc. should follow the test directory of the new instrument. If you are adding or deleting tests, you will need to send in a form to CMS to inform them of the change. You will need to receive the CMS approval back before you can put added tests into service.

If you are adding tests and anticipate a significant increase in test volume with the new instrument, you may need to hire additional lab staff. In my experience adding a few tests will not increase test volume enough to justify new hiring.

The new instrument will need to have routine maintenance. Usually the instrument maintenance scheduling and documentation fall on the section supervisor of the section where the instrument is located. In a few labs the Lab Supervisor is tasked with this.

The staff must be trained on how to operate the new analyzer. Usually this training is done by the Service Rep after he or she has done all other work in preparing to set the new analyzer in service. If the testing is particularly complicated, one or more of your techs may be asked to go to off-site training. This is typically held at the headquarters of the company that made the analyzer, but the training can also be from a third party.

There are limited numbers of seats at the off-site training, typically only 2 or 3 seats. This off-site training is typically seen as a free vacation by the junior techs. The senior techs typically see it as a prestigious perk. The distribution of these seats can be very contentious. For the most part, you are obligated to send the section supervisor of the section where the analyzer will be located. The other one or two seats are up for grabs, but usually go to the next highest ranking techs in the section where the analyzer will be located.

Any tech that wants to go to the off-site training and is not chosen will be very upset. Be prepared to give something of significant value to the techs passed up for the off-site training - raises, bonuses, etc. It is not uncommon for techs to threaten to quit when they find out they have not been chosen for the off-site training. I have seen at least one tech leave for a different company when passed up in this manner.

A peace offering given in appeasement is known as a "sop". In a few places in this book, I will indicate situations where something of value should be offered to employees passed up for promotion, made to work in sections of lab they don't prefer to work in, made to work excessive overtime, etc. In each instance this is an example of a sop.

Immediately before the new equipment is put in service, the hospital's information technology office should be called in to interface the new instrument with the hospital computer system. Look at how the reports will appear when testing is done on the new instrument. Is the reference range displayed? Is the report neat and easy to read? Once you have this worked out, you are ready to go live with the new instrument.

Initially the old instrument and new instrument run alongside each other, until the old instrument uses up all its remaining supplies and reagents. This allows time to make sure the new instrument is running properly.

After a few weeks to a few months the old instrument will use up all its remaining reagents and supplies. If the new instrument is working well without problems, the old instrument is then surveyed out (decommissioned and disposed of). The old instrument's procedure manual is retired to the retired procedure file.

The new instrument will have a schedule of preventive maintenance set by the manufacturer. It is very important to follow this schedule. Failure to follow this schedule can void the warranty.

The new analyzer will come with a list of things to avoid, which if done to the analyzer will void the warranty. Examples include putting a different manufacturer's parts into the analyzer, allowing anyone else but the Service Rep to put parts into the analyzer, using tap water in a analyzer that requires distilled water, etc.

It is imperative that you and the lab techs that operate the analyzer know what is not allowed by the manufacturer. You do not want to void the warranty as that would cause a whole series of problems. In my experience, no insurance company would ever insure an analyzer with a voided warranty. No bank would ever lend you money using that analyzer as collateral which means the lease might have to be unwound.

Chapter 8 – How to put a new test onto an existing analyzer

Putting a new test onto an existing analyzer is similar to putting a new piece of equipment into commission but involves fewer steps and fewer analytes.

Let's say that you have a chemistry instrument that is capable of doing serum radon levels, but there really hasn't been much interest in this particular test. You get one test request per year, and you send it out.

Then a few studies come out linking serum radon levels to lung cancer. The health news media runs huge numbers of stories. Suddenly your lab is swamped with specimens for serum radon testing, and sending out dozens per week. The pulmonologist tells you that given the recent journal articles, he will be ordering serum radon levels dozens of times per week forever.

In this scenario, if you can do the test on your existing equipment, you are pretty much obligated to implement the test in house. Here's how to do it.

The first thing to do is order the testing reagents, calibrators, and enroll in PT. As mentioned above the Lab Manager is responsible for all lab ordering of materials. When the reagents and calibrators arrive, do the calibration and the calibration verification.

Use 20 split specimens to correlate your instrument. If anyone else in the vicinity is doing the test, split 20 specimens, test a split in house, and send a split to the other lab. Correlate your equipment with their equipment. If no one else in the vicinity is doing the test, split 20 specimens, test a split in house, send the other part of the split specimens to the reference lab, and correlate the results. A correlation coefficient higher than 0.95 is preferable but not required.

Adopt the manufacturer's reference range, critical values and Analytic Measurement Range (AMR). Running linearity is desirable but not essential.

Once you enroll in PT you will receive the PT once every 4 months. You can start doing the test in-house after you have enrolled in PT, but before the first PT event has arrived. You will need to send in a form to CMS to inform them of the added in-house test.

Chapter 9 – How to deal with analyzer breakdowns

If a test is critical, you are going to have at least 2 analyzers capable of assaying that analyte. Typically, one is used as the primary analyzer, doing most of the work, and the other is a backup, used only when the first analyzer goes down or is taken down for maintenance. In a well funded hospital lab, the existing analyzers are replaced with new analyzers typically every 5 to 7 years, so that the analyzers never get old enough to have frequent breakdowns. In a well funded hospital it is extremely rare for both analyzers to go down at the same time.

In my 23 years experience in Pathology and Lab Medicine I have worked at two very underfunded municipal hospitals. Both put off purchases of new analyzers until the old analyzers were well past their usual lifespan and having frequent breakdowns. I requested new analyzers on several occasions. On each occasion the analyzers were budgeted for, but later the budget was readjusted with the money for the analyzers reallocated for an urgent need elsewhere in the same hospital. As a result, I have seen almost every type of analyzer breakdown imaginable. The list includes:

1. The analyzer gives off error codes and refuses to do anything.
2. The analyzer is out of control and can't be brought back into control.
3. The hospital has not paid its bills to the vendors. The vendors have put the hospital on "credit hold" meaning that they will not send more reagents until the prior shipments are paid for. The hospital lab has run out of reagents for that analyte.
4. Reagents have been paid for and are in transit, but the new reagents do not arrive before the existing reagents run out.
5. The analyzer refuses to boot because the motherboard has been damaged/destroyed by an electric power surge or outage.
6. Every moving part (arm, belt, etc.) is subject to wear and breakdown
7. The software is subject to viruses, corruption, hard drive failure, etc.

If one analyzer goes down, there is some urgency in getting it fixed, since you dread having both analyzers down at the same time. As a Lab Director you will become very proficient at dealing with analyzer breakdowns if you have to deal with them frequently. The same applies for all other lab disciplines - I spent a year at a Veteran's Hospital and became extremely good at looking at prostate biopsies. I spent 16 years in an underfunded municipal hospital and became extremely good at dealing with analyzer breakdowns.

When an analyzer breaks down, the bench level tech will be the first one to try to fix it. The first thing to do is to diagnose the analyzer's problems. The analyzer may give symptoms such as an error message, funny noise, restricted motion on an arm, etc.

If it is giving off an error code, look up the error code in the analyzer's owner's manual. An analyzer has an owner's manual which is usually stored in a binder in the same area as the procedure manuals. Look up the error code. It will give you a description of the problem, usually with suggested fixes. A common problem is plugged tubes. This usually gives off an error message related to high pressure in the tubing as the analyzer tries to pump fluids through the blocked tube.

If the problem is a funny noise, or restricted motion on the swing arm, this indicates a mechanical problem. This should prompt an immediate call to the hospital's BioMedical Department.

If the only problem is that the analyzer is out of control the tech can usually solve this on his or her own. The tech will first try rerunning the control. If the first or second rerun is in control, discard the original control results and accept the rerun control results.

If the two reruns are still out of control the tech will then try recalibration, ordering new controls, and sending a split of your existing controls to an outside lab for testing to see if your controls have deteriorated. If this does not fix the problem the next step is to call the analyzer manufacturer's headquarters.

The manufacturer's corporate headquarters should have techs available 24 hours a day 7 days a week that specialize in handling these sorts of trouble calls. These techs are usually very helpful in guiding you through the corrective process over the phone. If the analyzer still can't be brought back into control with their assistance, it usually means the analyzer has developed a hardware problem. The Service Rep is called and asked to come in person to fix the analyzer.

The tech must be very careful not to release any patient test results generated on an analyzer that is out of control. Those results are assumed to be erroneous and are discarded. If you have two analyzers, use the one that is in control until such time as the other analyzer is brought back into control. If both analyzers are out of control, the specimens must be sent out, or stored until such time that one analyzer or the other is brought back into control

If the analyzer refuses to boot and the power light does not come on check the electric cord, circuit breaker, universal power supply, and/or any special electric supply for the analyzer.

If the power light comes on, but the analyzer does not boot properly, or freezes up and reboots in an endless cycle, this usually indicates a software problem. This should prompt an immediate call to the hospital's Information Services or BioMed department, whichever handles the analyzer software issues.

If the bench tech, and anyone called in by the bench tech, is unable to fix the analyzer they call in the section supervisor who in turn calls in the Lab Supervisor. Each person called in will try to diagnose the problem. BioMed will come and open up the analyzer, such that all the tubes and wires will be visible. They will visually inspect to try to identify the problem.

The next step is a conference call to the Service Rep. This conference call will occur in the same room as the analyzer. The Service Rep typically gives instructions to the BioMed personnel "Try flushing the serum radon line and tell me what happens". BioMed will respond over the phone "we tried flushing the line and the flow is good. It was not blocked". This series of diagnostic maneuvers will continue until the problem is identified.

After diagnosing the problem, you have to fix it. If you are lucky the analyzer will have a problem that can be fixed easily, such as a blocked tube. If the problem is a broken part BioMed will try to fix the part.

If BioMed can't fix the part, you need to have a new part flown in. It is very unlikely that anyone in the same state as you has the part available. Everyone with this analyzer needs that particular part for their analyzer to work. You would need to find a lab that has the exact same equipment as you, and has enough backup analyzers that they could take one analyzer down to give you the part. In my experience, this never happens.

In this situation, you are going to have to order the part from the manufacturer and it will have to be flown in. The manufacturer usually doesn't allow anyone but their Service Rep to put a new part into their analyzer. Thus you will have to wait for the Service Rep to arrive to put the part in. The analyzer will be down until both the part and the Service Rep have arrived. In the remote places where I have been working, that could be 5 days or more.

You will have a very nervous 5 days waiting for the part and Service Rep to arrive. If you are lucky you will get the malfunctioning analyzer up and running before the other analyzer can break down. If the other analyzer breaks down before the first one can be fixed, follow the diagnostic steps above for both analyzers. In this situation it is imperative that you get one analyzer or the other up and running as soon as possible.

If both analyzers break down at the same time you cannot do an essential test. You are in a world of hurt and you have to improvise. Your patient's lives depend on you being able to do the test. You will be scrambling, and you will improvise any way you can.

Once while I was working at an underfunded, remote municipal hospital both CBC analyzers went down at the same time. One had its motherboard fried by an electric power surge, the other needed a part. The parts could be flown in within about 3 days. However, the Service Rep was in Singapore on a trouble call there and it would be at least 5 days before the Service Rep would arrive. There was a military hospital in that municipality, but it was a 45 minute drive to get there. This is how we handled the CBCs while the analyzers were down:

1. Any patient so critical as to be unable to wait the added 45 minutes drive time would get a spun crit. The tech would make a slide and do a microscopic platelet estimate, WBC estimate and manual differential. These would be called to the patient's Attending Physician as STAT results. The tube of blood was then sent out for the automated CBC.

2. Any patient that could wait the added 45 minute drive time had their tube of blood couriered over to the military hospital for a routine automated CBC.

The same underfunded, remote municipal hospital had ABG analyzer breakdowns. This hospital was doing its ABG's on Cobas analyzers. Both went down at the same time due to a reagent outage. This happened on a Saturday morning with the reagents in transit by air freight due to arrive Sunday night, about 36 hours later. This hospital lab borrowed an Abbot I-stat from the military hospital in the same municipality. This was done as an "emergency" borrow which would need the Admiral's approval when he arrived to work on Monday. The Admiral arrived to work Monday morning and disapproved of the military hospital's lending of the Abbot I-stat. By this time the reagents had arrived for the Cobas analyzers.

I must confess, this episode was the only instance in my career where a laboratory I headed was not able to follow CMS rules. The Cobas ABG analyzers went down in the hospital where I worked. There were 8 patients in ICU on ventilators. These patients needed ABG's at least daily and some as often as every 8 hours. Some or all of them could die if they didn't get ABG's. The only option is to borrow the Abbot I-stat from the military hospital to do the ABG testing. The testing was done without doing any of the necessary work described above for setting a new methodology into place (correlation, calibration, etc.). We could not do this after the fact, since the military hospital demanded the return of the Abbott I-stat analyzer the next working day.

The tech doing the testing manually entered the ABG test results into the hospital computer, and verified them as if they were done on the Cobas, when in fact they were not, they were done on a borrowed Abbot I-stat.

The CMS inspector did not catch this at the next inspection. This could have been caught in two ways. First, test results were generated on a day for which we had not done controls on the Cobas ABG analyzers. Second, results were present in the hospital computer that were not present in the Cobas analyzers. It would take a very astute inspector to notice this, and luckily the CMS inspector missed this at the next inspection. If the inspector had caught this, both the lab and I would have been in deep trouble.

I can tell these stories now that I am more or less retired. My experiences may have been unique. Most other Lab Directors work at better funded hospitals that are able to replace analyzers earlier in their lifespan, before they enter the phase of repeated breakdowns.

As a Lab Director, make sure that all the equipment in your lab is properly maintenanced and in good working order. You do not want to find yourself in situations similar to those described above. At the time these events were gut-wrenching; and even now, many years later, they are an unpleasant memory.

Chapter 10 – How to read a linearity proficiency test report

I have referenced linearity a number of times in prior chapters. It is very similar to Analytic Measurement Range (AMR). CLIA has requirements for AMR but is silent on linearity, so linearity tends to take a backseat to AMR.

Although CLIA has no requirement for linearity proficiency testing, most labs will test linearity twice a year. Linearity PT is particularly associated with chemistry analyzers but is also done in hematology. As a Lab Director you will need to know how to read a linearity proficiency testing event.

Here is an example of a recent linearity PT event on an older analyzer.

	EVALUATION ORIGINAL	Chemistry/Lipid/Enzyme Calibration Verification/Linearity Executive Summary		
Analyte	Calibration Verification		Linearity Evaluation	Page #
Albumin g/dL	Verified from 1.40 to 8.50		Linear from 1.40 to 8.50	2 - 3
Calcium mg/dL	Verified from 6.80 to 18.65		Linear from 6.80 to 18.65	4 - 5
Chloride mmol/L	Verified from 56.0 to 188.0		Linear from 56.0 to 188.0	6 - 7
CO2 mmol/L	***		Linear from 6.05 to 34.65	8
Creatinine mg/dL	Verified from 0.300 to 31.000		Linear from 0.300 to 31.000	9 - 10
Glucose mg/dL	Verified from 19.0 to 720.0		Linear from 19.0 to 720.0	11 - 12
Iron µg/dL	Verified from 12.5 to 850.0		Linear from 12.5 to 850.0	13 - 14
Magnesium mg/dL	Verified from 0.50 to 9.65		Linear from 0.50 to 9.65	15 - 16
Phosphorus mg/dL	Verified from 0.70 to 13.45		Linear from 0.70 to 13.45	17 - 18
Potassium mmol/L	Verified from 1.60 to 9.30		Linear from 1.60 to 9.30	19 - 20
Total Protein g/dL	Verified from 1.65 to 10.35		Linear from 1.65 to 10.35	21 - 22
Sodium mmol/L	*Verified from 91.5 to 173.0		Linear from 91.5 to 193.5	23 - 24
Urea Nitrogen (BUN) mg/dL	Verified from 2.0 to 183.0		Linear from 2.0 to 183.0	25 - 26
Uric Acid mg/dL	Verified from 0.90 to 24.35		Linear from 0.90 to 24.35	27 - 28
Direct Bilirubin mg/dL	Verified from 2.30 to 10.30		Linear from 2.30 to 10.30	29 - 30
Total Bilirubin mg/dL	Verified from 0.00 to 23.00		Linear from 0.00 to 23.00	31 - 32
Cholesterol mg/dL	Verified from 54.0 to 548.5		*Linear from 54.0 to 466.0	33 - 34
Triglyceride mg/dL	Verified from 20.0 to 622.0		Linear from 20.0 to 622.0	35 - 36
HDL Cholesterol mg/dL	**Different**		Linear from 5.0 to 29.0	37 - 38
ALT (SGPT) U/L	*Verified from 174.0 to 926.5		Linear from 23.5 to 926.5	39 - 40
Alkaline Phosphatase U/L	Verified from 49.0 to 1737.5		Linear from 49.0 to 1737.5	41 - 42
Amylase U/L	Verified from 25.0 to 758.0		Linear from 25.0 to 758.0	43 - 44
AST (SGOT) U/L	Verified from 11.0 to 938.5		Linear from 11.0 to 938.5	45 - 46
CK-2 (CK MB)-Mass ng/mL	Verified from 30.70 to 230.60		Linear from 30.70 to 230.60	47 - 48
Creatine Kinase U/L	Verified from 25.0 to 2119.0		Linear from 25.0 to 2119.0	49 - 50
GGT U/L	Verified from 19.0 to 1048.5		Linear from 19.0 to 1048.5	51 - 52
LD U/L	*Verified from 398.5 to 2083.0		Linear from 49.0 to 2083.0	53 - 54
Lipase U/L	Verified from 92.5 to 1358.5		Linear from 92.5 to 1358.5	55 - 56

Note: For results of Different, see the Calibration Verification Troubleshooting Guide and Investigation Checklist.

* This range does not include all reported specimens. Review your results to determine if excluded specimens reveal possible analytical problems.

*** No Peer Group

Reviewed by_____ Date_____

Notice that HDL cholesterol has failed linearity. On an older analyzer that is showing its age, it is not uncommon to fail linearity on one or more analyte. As mentioned in a prior chapter, if the instrument becomes non-linear for any analyte this could be an early warning sign that you are having problems with that particular test. The linearity tends to go out first, before the test goes out of control. As with all other problems, follow the corrective action procedure outlined in Chapter 5.

You are probably starting to notice by now that every time something goes wrong, I refer to the corrective action procedure, like a broken record playing the same note over and over. The fact of the matter is that the corrective action procedure is about the only thing you can do to correct a quality control failure on an analyzer. The only alternative would be to follow the analyzer breakdown procedure, but that procedure wouldn't be as applicable for failed linearity or other failed PT.

The carbon dioxide has three asterisks in the calibration verification field. At the bottom, the three asterisks indicates there is no peer group. No peer group means that no other lab is using the same particular combination of equipment and methodology you are using. In my experience, when you have no peer group it means you are the last lab using that equipment. In this circumstance your equipment is outdated and the manufacturer will likely soon stop supporting it forcing you to use a newer methodology.

When there is no peer group, you have to look in the accompanying participant summary to see what the intended answers were. If you were acceptably close to the intended result, make a handwritten note to that effect on the above page. If you were too far away from the intended result, make a corrective action.

Here is the sodium linearity:

EVALUATION ORIGINAL	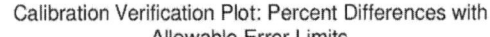 Chemistry/Lipid/Enzyme Calibration Verification/Linearity Sodium mmol/L Calibration Verification Evaluation

Evaluation Result: Verified from 91.5 to 173.0

Peer Instrument:
Peer Method:

Allowable Error: 2.5% or 2 mmol/L, whichever is greater

Specimen	Assay 1	Assay 2	Your Mean	Peer Mean	Peer N	Difference	Allowable Error
LN-28	92	91	91.5	90.8	43	0.8%	± 2.5%
LN-29	111	111	111.0	110.1	43	0.8%	± 2.5%
LN-30	132	132	132.0	129.4	43	2.0%	± 2.5%
LN-31	152	152	152.0	149.1	43	1.9%	± 2.5%
LN-32	173	173	173.0	168.8	42	2.5%	± 2.5%
LN-33	194	193	193.5	186.9	41	3.5%	± 2.5%
LN-34	> 214	> 214		206.9	26		± 2.5%

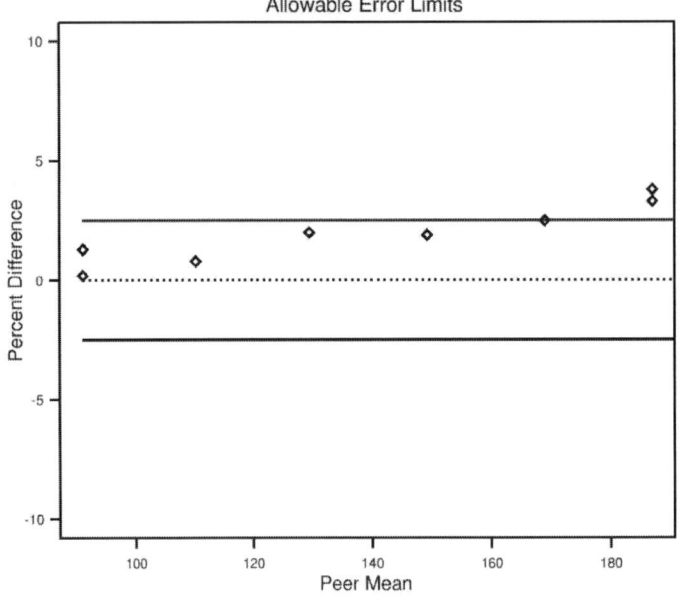

Peer Results Summary Table   Your evaluation may not be included in the peer results.   Peer Group Size: 43

	Calibration Verification		Linearity Evaluation		
Range	% Verified	% Different	% Linear	% Nonlinear	% Imprecise
LN-28 - 34	44.2	9.3	53.5	0.0	0.0
LN-28 - 33	32.6	4.7	37.2	0.0	4.7
LN-28 - 32	4.7	0.0	2.3	0.0	0.0
LN-28 - 31	4.7	0.0	2.3	0.0	0.0

The sodium passed the five lover levels, but failed the most extreme high level, reporting greater than 214 mmol/L on a specimen that should have reported 209 mmol/L. As a result, the linear range for sodium is 91.5 to 173 mmol/L. That is not a big problem. The reference range for serum sodium levels is between 135 and 145 mmol/L. Anything above 155 mmol/L is a critical high.

We will assume that the linearity PT material does not exceed the AMR of the analyzer. It wouldn't make sense for the linearity PT material to be outside the AMR of the analyzer. If it exceeded the AMR it would have to be diluted to be run on the analyzer. This would complicate things unnecessarily such that it isn't generally done for this type of PT.

Making the assumption the linearity PT material does not exceed the AMR of the analyzer, a corrective action might get this test back to being able to read extremely elevated serum sodium levels. Most people won't bother with a corrective action for this since it is not necessary to measure serum sodium at a concentration that is not compatible with life. However, as mentioned above, failed linearity can be an early warning sign of problems with a test, so I will do corrective action for this type of PT failure.

After you do the corrective action repeat the test for the specimen that failed if any of that specimen remains. If the result for that analyte is now in the expected range, you have just proven linearity for the entire AMR for that analyte. You can keep the same AMR as before, in this situation the AMR does not need to be adjusted.

Let's say we do the corrective action, but still fail on the sodium level of 209 mmol/L. This means our linear range is 91.5 to 173 mmol/L. We have to reduce our AMR accordingly. Anything above 173 mmol/L we report as "greater than 173 mmol/L" or dilute and repeat. If a living person really did have a serum sodium of 209 mmol/L, we could dilute the specimen, repeat the test and measure the sodium. Alternatively, we could report it as a "greater than 173 mmol/L" panic value. Either way, this is a critically high sodium level.

Next let's take a look at how we did on the cholesterol:

EVALUATION ORIGINAL	Chemistry/Lipid/Enzyme Calibration Verification/Linearity Cholesterol mg/dL Calibration Verification Evaluation

Evaluation Result: Verified from 54.0 to 548.5
Peer Instrument:
Peer Method:

Allowable Error: 4.5% or 3 mg/dL, whichever is greater

Specimen	Assay 1	Assay 2	Your Mean	Peer Mean	Peer N	Difference	Allowable Error
LN-41	< 29	< 29		29.2	76		± 3.0 mg/dL
LN-42	54	54	54.0	54.9	156	-0.9 mg/dL	± 3.0 mg/dL
LN-43	142	142	142.0	143.2	156	-0.8%	± 4.5%
LN-44	258	259	258.5	258.1	156	0.2%	± 4.5%
LN-45	363	363	363.0	362.3	156	0.2%	± 4.5%
LN-46	467	465	466.0	467.3	156	-0.3%	± 4.5%
LN-47	549	548	(548.5)	(549.1)	155	-0.1%	± 4.5%

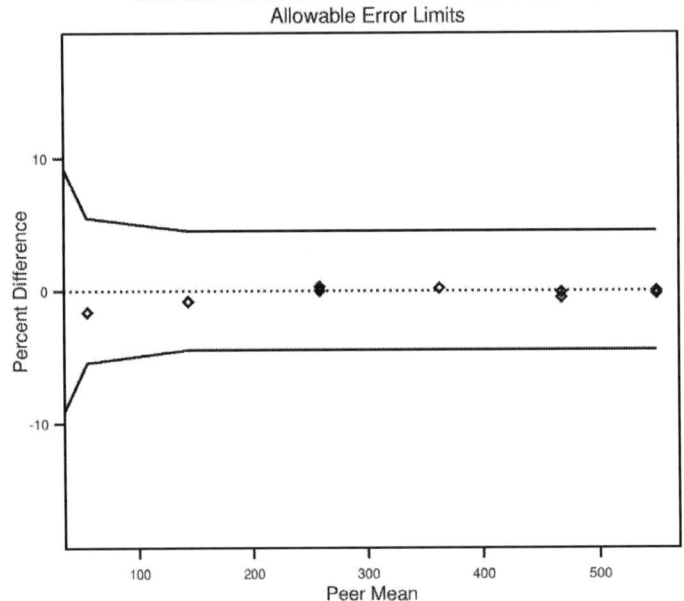

Peer Results Summary Table   Your evaluation may not be included in the peer results.   Peer Group Size: 156

Range	Calibration Verification		Linearity Evaluation		
	% Verified	% Different	% Linear	% Nonlinear	% Imprecise
LN-41 - 47	21.8	17.9	12.2	0.0	0.0
LN-41 - 46	3.8	0.0	32.7	0.0	0.0
LN-42 - 47	30.1	5.1	14.7	0.0	0.0
LN-41 - 45	1.3	0.0	1.3	0.0	1.3
LN-42 - 46	6.4	0.0	35.3	0.0	0.0
LN-43 - 47	8.3	0.0	0.0	0.0	0.0
LN-41 - 44	1.9	0.0	1.3	0.0	0.0
LN-42 - 45	0.6	0.0	1.3	0.0	0.0
LN-43 - 46	2.6	0.0	0.0	0.0	0.0

For LN-47 our mean is 548.5 mg/dL and the peer mean (i.e. everybody else in the world testing the same PT material using the same equipment and methodology) got an average of 549.1 mg/dL. We are off by about 0.1%. As far as I am concerned, we hit the bullseye. The next chart shows the cholesterol linearity.

| | EVALUATION ORIGINAL | | Chemistry/Lipid/Enzyme Calibration Verification/Linearity Cholesterol mg/dL Linearity Evaluation |

Evaluation Result: Linear from 54.0 to 466.0
Instrument:
Method:

Evaluation Type: Standard
Goal for Total Error (TE): 9%
Mean of Included Results: 256.7 mg/dL

Specimen	Assay 1	Assay 2	Your Mean	Best-fit Target	Relative Concentration
LN-41	< 29	< 29			0.000
LN-42	54	54	54.0	58.9	0.050
LN-43	142	142	142.0	141.3	0.200
LN-44	258	259	258.5	251.2	0.400
LN-45	363	363	363.0	361.1	0.600
LN-46	467	465	466.0	470.9	0.800
LN-47	549	548	548.5	580.8	1.000

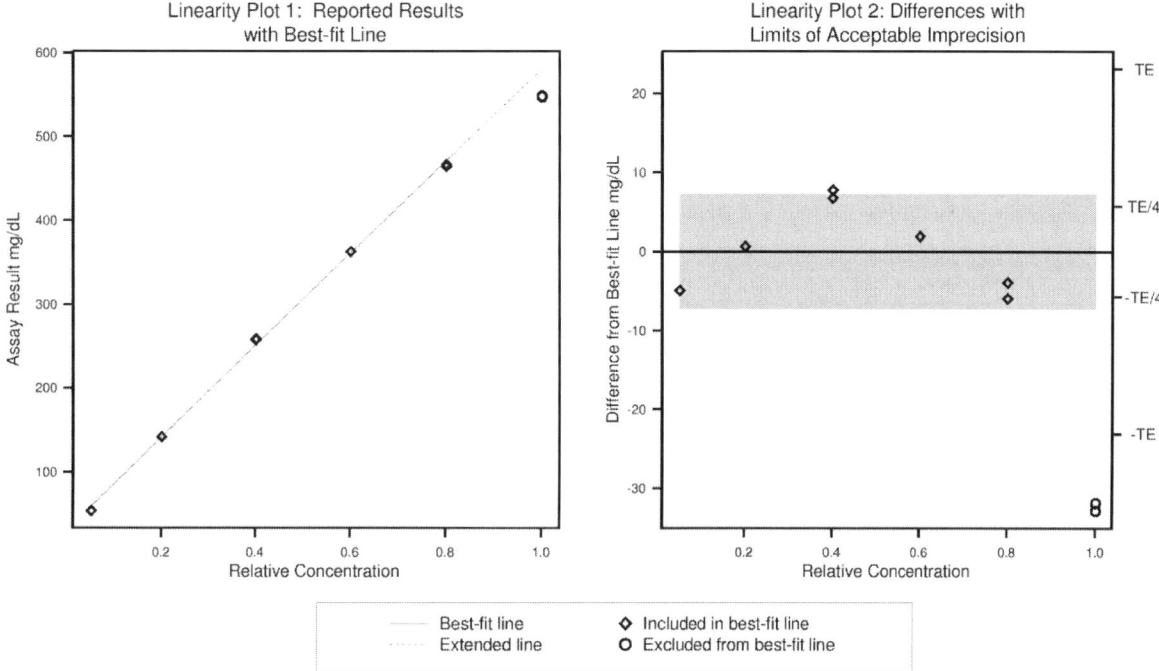

Your plot has one or more points within your linear range that fall outside of the shaded area. Since your evaluation is Linear, no remedial action is necessary.

Points can fall outside of the shaded area for two reasons:
1) an average is used to estimate imprecision, so many small differences can offset a few large differences, and
2) clinically insignificant nonlinearity (curved fit) can contribute to differences between your results and the best-fit straight line. Larger differences may be an early warning sign of nonlinearity, poor repeatability, or poor fit.

The cholesterol linearity graph falls away from a straight line for LN-47, the extreme high cholesterol. Our result is 548.5 md/dL however the best fit target is 580.8 mg/dL cholesterol. As far as I am concerned, we hit the bullseye with an average almost exactly the same as every other lab using the same equipment and method.

The manufacturer of the PT material thinks they spiked enough cholesterol into LN-47 that it should report 580.8 mg/dL cholesterol. However, every lab in existence using the same analyzer and method we are using reports 549 mg/dL cholesterol. I am suspicious that the problem is with the manufacturer of the PT material, and not with every analyzer in the world.

Let's give the benefit of the doubt to the PT maker. Every lab in the world using the same analyzer and same method we are using got the wrong result. Most chemistry tests are enzymatic or immunoassays, and at extreme high concentrations of the analyte most of the enzymes or antibodies used for testing are already saturated with analyte. In this range a +1 increase in the "true" analyte concentration may result in a less than +1 increase in the test result. Thus our linearity for cholesterol really is from 54.0 to 466.0 mg/dL.

Although the test is not linear at 549 mg/dL, our results are almost exactly the same as every other lab in the world using the same analyzer and method. The results are reproducible, both runs gave very close numbers. I would feel comfortable turning out cholesterol test results up to 549 mg/dL on this analyzer, since it is accurate, precise and reproducible. However, the CMS inspectors would likely object that the linearity of the analyzer has been exceeded, so I do not do this. Instead the AMR for cholesterol is set from 54.0 to 466.0 mg/dL.

Similar to the sodium testing discussed above, the cholesterol testing is in the same situation of reduced AMR upper limit. It is possible to dilute and rerun any specimen with a cholesterol over 466.0 mg/dL. The difference between 466 mg/dL and 549 mg/dL cholesterol is probably not that significant anyhow; they are both callable high values. The AMR of the test is set at the limits of linearity determined by this PT event from 54.0 to 466.0 mg/dL.

In this circumstance, doing a corrective action would likely be a futile maneuver. We have already hit the bullseye, reporting results within about 0.1% of every other lab in the world using the same analyzer and method. You really can't improve on this. Hence, a corrective action should not be able to accomplish anything.

Here is the linearity for HDL cholesterol.

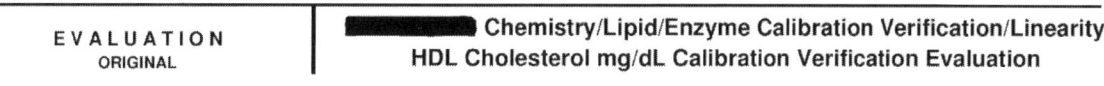

EVALUATION ORIGINAL	Chemistry/Lipid/Enzyme Calibration Verification/Linearity HDL Cholesterol mg/dL Calibration Verification Evaluation

Evaluation Result: Different
Your Instrument:
Your Method:
Peer Instrument:

Allowable Error: 10% or 2 mg/dL, whichever is greater

Specimen	Assay 1	Assay 2	Your Mean	Peer Mean	Peer N	Difference	Allowable Error
LN-41	< 4	< 4		4.2	128		± 2.0 mg/dL
LN-42	5	5	5.0	6.6	154	-1.6 mg/dL	± 2.0 mg/dL
LN-43	11	11	11.0	13.3	160	-2.3 mg/dL	± 2.0 mg/dL
LN-44	17	16	16.5	20.6	160	-19.9%	± 10.0%
LN-45	21	22	21.5	26.3	160	-18.3%	± 10.0%
LN-46	25	24	24.5	31.8	160	-23.0%	± 10.0%
LN-47	29	29	29.0	35.7	160	-18.8%	± 10.0%

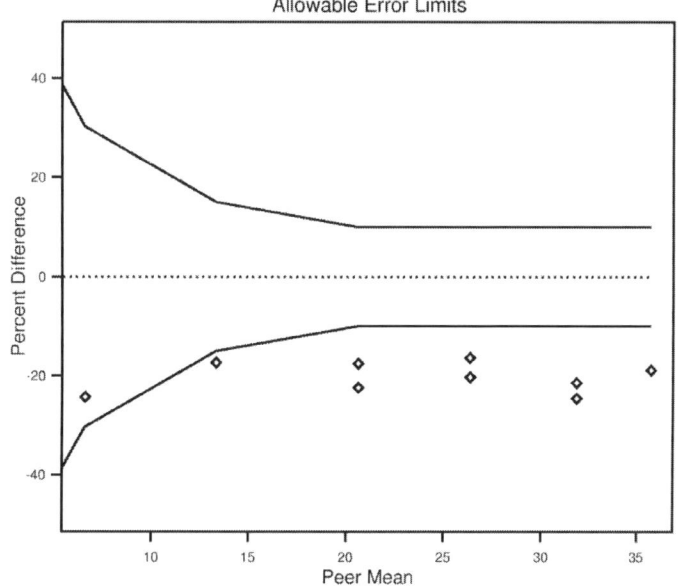

Calibration Verification Plot: Percent Differences with Allowable Error Limits

Peer Results Summary Table Your evaluation may not be included in the peer results. Peer Group Size: 160

Range	Calibration Verification		Linearity Evaluation		
	% Verified	% Different	% Linear	% Nonlinear	% Imprecise
LN-41 - 47	41.9	18.1	15.6	0.6	1.3
LN-41 - 46	5.6	0.0	31.9	0.0	0.0
LN-42 - 47	5.6	5.6	13.1	0.6	0.6
LN-41 - 45	6.3	0.0	18.8	0.0	0.0
LN-42 - 46	0.6	0.0	1.3	0.0	0.0
LN-43 - 47	5.0	1.9	3.8	0.0	0.0
LN-41 - 44	8.1	0.0	11.9	0.0	0.0
LN-42 - 45	0.6	0.0	0.6	0.0	0.0
LN-43 - 46	0.6	0.0	0.0	0.0	0.0

The HDL cholesterol linearity is quite a disaster. Every result has a huge negative bias. You will need to do a corrective action for the HDL cholesterol. Be careful to look through the recent controls, to make sure this test really is in control. Given how badly it failed linearity, it is surprising that the controls were in.

The corrective action was carried out for the HDL cholesterol linearity given above. There was no problem with the testing; the problem was that the wrong box had been filled in for method code on the form returned to the proficiency testing provider. This one small mistake in filling out the form caused our HDL cholesterol results to be measured against the results generated by a different methodology on a different analyzer. In other words, the linearity shown above is comparing apples to oranges; our results using our method are not directly comparable to the results generated by a different method or analyzer.

One has to pay attention to the smallest details. The smallest mistake in filling out the proficiency testing form caused us to badly fail HDL cholesterol linearity. In this case, we informed the proficiency testing provider of our mistake, asked them to re-grade the HDL cholesterol, and send us a new proficiency testing evaluation, so as to have a passing linearity in the file to show the inspector.

Chapter 11 – How to write a policy and/or procedure

A policy is a statement of intent. It is usually dogmatic, broad and vague, stated in very general terms. For example: "The Lab will uphold quality patient testing". "The Lab will not tolerate unacceptable practices".

A procedure is a written document used to implement policy. It usually lists step by step instructions on how to do things, similar to a cookbook. Deviations from the lab's procedures can only occur under extreme circumstances, and usually require permission from the Lab Director or other authority.

The "procedures" in the typical lab procedure manual are really a mix of both policy and procedure. When I say "procedure" in this book, I am referring to the written documentation in the typical lab manual. Everyone refers to this as "procedure" even though it really is a mix of both policy and procedure.

The original copies of all lab procedures are usually kept in a secure location. This is usually the Lab Secretary's computer, provided that the secretary's office is locked at night and the secretary's computer is password protected. The Lab Secretary will have to retype all changed procedures once every 2 years in the run-up to the CMS or CAP inspection, so it makes sense that the procedures should be kept on his or her computer.

The Lab Secretary is usually given an unofficial designation as "manual guardian", "procedure protector", etc. It is his or her responsibility to maintain the integrity of the procedure manuals. Be sure to emphasize how important this is and not to allow any unauthorized individuals access to the procedure manuals, secretary's computer, etc.

One often overlooked point is backing up the procedures. I have seen one hard drive crash wipe out hundreds of pages of procedure manual. It is imperative that you make backups at least monthly. I prefer optical media such as CD-R and DVD-R, however others prefer thumb drives, etc. The procedure manuals are thousands of pages; however, text documents are quite compact in terms of computer bytes. The entirety of the lab's procedure manuals should fit on one DVD-R or thumb drive.

The Lab Secretary's computer is not accessible to the lab techs but CLIA requires that the testing personnel have access to the procedures in the testing area. Usually this is accomplished by making a hardcopy printout of the procedures and putting them in multiple large 3 ring binders in each section of lab.

This is less commonly done by having copies available on the computers in the work area of lab. If you are going to keep the procedures "paperless" you have to be very careful that all techs are able to access the procedures in the testing area. If the CMS inspectors see that your procedures are "paperless" they are bound to ask several techs to look up several procedures. If even one tech can't find one procedure your lab will be cited. This is a favorite citation of the CMS inspectors. Hence, in my experience, you are better off with multiple 3 ring binders.

The reviewing and updating of each lab section's procedures is typically the responsibility of the section supervisor. The Chemistry supervisor has the most knowledge of Chemistry procedures compared to anyone else in lab. The Blood Bank supervisor has the most knowledge of Blood Bank procedures compared to anyone else in lab, etc. It makes sense that they should oversee the work on the procedures for their areas. The general lab procedures are reviewed and updated by the Lab Supervisor.

After being downloaded, written or changed by the section supervisor, the procedure may or may not be signed off by the Lab Supervisor and is always signed by the Lab Director. Both CMS and CAP require that the Lab Director approve of any new or changed procedure in lab. CAP requires the Lab Director to sign all procedures once every 2 years, but CMS does not require this biannual review.

Lab procedures are usually written in simple easy to understand language that tells the tech how to do the testing in a one step at a time, cookbook manner. The procedure has to be understood by the least intelligent tech in lab, so the language tends to be simple and clear. The procedure has to reflect what you are doing in real life and what you are doing in real life has to be documented in the procedure.

If the way your lab does things changes, even a little, you have to change the procedure in the manual. The change is typically written into the hardcopy printout of the procedure present in the work area. It must be signed and dated by the Lab Director in order to be valid.

For example, one of the citations on my most recent CMS inspection involved the procedure for urinalysis. The vendor supplying lab had switched dipsticks from one manufacturer to another. The testing was the same, the interpretation was the same, but the name of the manufacturer switched. My lab had the name of the old manufacturer written into the procedure manual. The inspector caught this and cited us.

Once every 2 years in the run-up to the CMS or CAP inspection, these 3 ring binders are brought into the Lab Secretary's Office. Any written changes are then typed into the original copy of the procedure on the Lab Secretary's computer. The re-typed procedures are then printed out, signed by the Lab Director and put in the 3 ring binders as part of the preparation for the next CMS or CAP inspection.

Depending on how many procedures have changed, this could be a huge amount of work on the part of the Lab Secretary. Make sure to give the Lab Secretary something of value (overtime, comp time, etc.) in exchange. As mentioned previously, a peace offering given in appeasement is known as a "sop".

As Lab Director, you want all testing to meet regulatory requirements. The techs would prefer the easiest procedure possible. If the lab is adding a new test or modifying an existing test, you will likely be making more work for the techs. As Lab Director you may have to do some negotiation with the techs who will be doing the testing. It is best to offer them something of value (overtime, comp time, etc.) in exchange. This is yet another example of a sop.

Once the procedure has been signed by the Lab Director it goes in the procedure manual. You have to make sure that all the techs are aware of the new or changed procedure. This usually entails calling all the techs into one room at the same time and informing them of the new or changed procedure. It is best to buy pizza or otherwise serve food at this meeting. The techs may be very unhappy that you are making more work for them.

A procedure is needed for every test offered in lab. The lab also needs to have procedures for calibration, verification of calibration, running controls, corrective action to take when controls are out, a description of the course of action to take if a test system becomes inoperable, quality assurance, etc.

The procedure for each test should include requirements for patient preparation; specimen collection and processing, criteria for specimen acceptability and rejection, instructions for step-by-step performance of the procedure, interpretation of results, preparation of all materials used in testing, the reportable range for test results, limitations in the test methodology including interfering substances, reference intervals (normal values), critical results (panic values) and the laboratory's system for entering results in the patient record and reporting patient results. The reference for this is 42 CFR§ 493.1251.

In the typical hospital lab this amount of documentation can run into thousands of pages. Typing that amount of documentation would take an eternity and would be impractical. Most labs get their procedure manuals from the test manufacturer or download the procedures from the internet. Another source for procedures is nearby hospital labs using the same equipment.

As a Lab Director, you will not be writing procedures, but will be reviewing them for accuracy. Things to check are:

1. Oversights and skipped steps are a common problem. Is the procedure complete? Does one step lead to the next, or is something missing in between?
2. Is it easy to understand? Is the least intelligent tech in lab going to have a hard time reading and understanding it?
3. Could a lab tech new to this workplace read the procedure, and do the test without supervision and without asking for help?
4. Does it reflect what is being done in real life? If a specific manufacturer is named, are we still using that manufacturer?
5. Has anything changed since the time the procedure was written?

If you are not satisfied with the procedure, you can change it as you see fit. Keep in mind that the techs will have to follow the procedure exactly. Try not to put anything onerous in the procedure.

Below is an example of a procedure, the Blood Bank Emergency Release of Blood procedure.

MY LAB
BLOOD BANK PROCEDURE MANUAL

CATEGORY: **OPERATIONS/MANAGEMENT**	CODE: **3144**
SUBJECT: **Emergency Release of Blood**	EFFECTIVE: **12/2013**
RESPONSIBLE DEPARTMENT/DESIGNEE: **BLOOD BANK**	PAGE: 1 of 3

POLICY: Experienced personnel are available in the Blood Bank on a 24-hour basis to assist with the provision of blood and blood components during emergencies. Only Blood Bank employees are allowed access to the blood inventory, or are permitted to issue blood for transfusion.

Procedure to request blood during an emergency:

1. Call Blood Bank at extension XXXX

2. Describe the urgency of the situation. "The ER/OR/ICU has a patient with an emergency need for transfusion".

3. Provide the patient's name and medical record number. For multiple patients with unknown names, see the Mass Casualty Disaster procedure.

4. Indicate the blood component and amount required. Indicate how quickly it is needed - immediate, 10 minutes, 45 minutes etc.

5. Provide the number and name of the ordering physician

6. Indicate the location of the patient

7. Blood Bank will read back orders and patient identifiers to assure accuracy.

The Blood Bank will check if it already has crossmatched blood for the patient. If crossmatched blood is not currently available, the Blood Bank can then determine the extent to which compatibility testing can be performed. As the amount of compatibility testing decreases, the possible risk of transfusing incompatible blood increases. Depending on the availability of a specimen and current status of testing blood may be released as:

1. **Uncrossmatched red blood cells:**
    - Available immediately

- Should only be requested in situations where the transfusion cannot wait 10 minutes for patient typing.
- Type O-negative blood is the universal donor blood. It is rare and hard to obtain. It should only be used in life-or-death emergencies.

2. **Type specific blood:**
   - Available after typing the patient (10 minutes required for typing).
   - Should be used in situations where transfusion can wait 10 minutes but cannot wait about 45 minutes

3. **Full cross match blood:**
   - The full crossmatch requires about 45 minutes to complete.
   - A fully cross matched unit has the least risk of causing a transfusion reaction.

4. **Least Incompatible blood:**
   - In a patient with an unexpected antibody, it may not be possible to obtain a cross match negative unit.
   - This type of transfusion comes with significant risks of a transfusion reaction. It should only be given if the benefits outweigh the risks.
   - The patient should be informed of the risks of this type of transfusion.

Release of Blood:

1. The nurse or other authorized person will come to Blood Bank.

2. The release of blood will follow the same procedure as described in the Issue and Release of Blood and Blood Components procedure.

3. For uncrossmatched blood, the cross match will be completed after the transfusion. The patient's Attending Physician will be notified promptly if the cross match is found to be positive.

4. For least incompatible units, the antibody identification and donor unit typing will be completed after the transfusion. The patient's Attending Physician will be notified promptly of the results.

REVIEWED AND APPROVED BY:

_____   _____
Blood Bank Supervisor   Date

_____   _____
Lab Supervisor   Date

_____   _____
Lab Director   Date

**Reviewed Last
(Date and Initial)**

_____

_____

_____

For each procedure, the date of creation and each date of modification is typed into the procedure. After a procedure is no longer needed, it is retired to the retired procedure folder. The retirement date is logged in the retired procedure logbook. CLIA and CAP mandate that retired procedures should be kept at least two years. In my experience the retention of retired procedures is indefinite. They tend to sit forever in a filing cabinet in the office area, never to be disposed of, unless there is a desperate need for space in the filing cabinet.

Chapter 12 – Quality Assurance, complaints, incident reports and root cause analysis

CLIA requires that all labs have a Quality Assurance (QA) program. In most larger labs there is a QA coordinator who takes care of all the QA work. I have spent most of my career working in small labs in remote areas which do not have a QA coordinator. In the absence of a QA coordinator, the work falls on the Lab Supervisor and the Lab Director.

The usual list of QA indicators to measure include:

1. Greater than 90% of STAT tests turned around within 1 hour
2. 100% of tests marked "Routine" turned around (or canceled) within one day (24 hours) of ordering.
3. 100% of tested specimens properly labeled as to patient name, identification, etc. All unidentified specimens rejected by lab and not tested.
4. Corrected (modified) test results
5. 100% of specimens are acceptable (all lipemic, hemolyzed specimens rejected if lipemia/hemolysis will affect test results).
6. 100% of critical values (panic values) called to the provider.
7. Complaints and/or incident reports involving Lab.
8. Inpatient AM lab draw turn around time
9. Blood culture contamination rate
10. Crossmatch:transfusion ratio below 1.5

CLIA is silent on what exactly your QA program has to measure. In theory, you could pick only one criterion from the above list, measure it, and you would have a QA program. In reality, most labs pick about 5 of the above 10 QA indicators. If you pick the entire list, you are going to be working very hard. You are not limited to this list. You can measure anything you want to in lab and call it QA.

Although CLIA is silent on what a lab's QA program must measure, CMS places requirements on the hospital as a whole. These state that the hospital must develop, implement, and maintain an effective, ongoing, hospital-wide, data-driven quality assessment and performance improvement program. There must be an ongoing program that shows measurable improvement in indicators for which there is evidence that it will improve health outcomes and identify and reduce medical errors. The hospital must set priorities for its performance improvement activities that focus on high-risk, high-volume, or problem-prone areas. The reference is 42 CFR § 482.21.

Thus, if you are in a hospital lab you will be mandated to do this as part of the hospital-wide QA program. If you are in an outpatient lab there is no specific requirement on what your QA program should measure. Either way, you can pick any 5 of the above list of 10 QA indicators, and you've got your QA program started.

You need to set criteria, usually expressed in terms of percent or ratio, that is considered passing for each of these QA indicators. You should document the significance of the indicator. In other words, what is the impact on patient care of passing or failing this QA indicator. If you know at the start that you are not passing for that QA indicator, you should set a goal or target with an explanation of what you are trying to achieve and why.

For patient safety indicators, only 0% is acceptable (i.e. no patient falls in lab). For other QA indicators the CMS has no set criteria. The suggestion is that your QA numbers should be comparable to similar hospitals elsewhere. In other words, you can ask similar sized hospital labs in the region what their QA indicators are and what they consider to be passing.

Laboratory testing can be divided into three analytical phases. The preanalytic phase is everything that occurs before the testing – identifying the patient by wristband, putting the correct patient's bar-code label on the tubes, etc. The analytic phase is the testing. The postanalytic phase occurs after the test – reporting the correct patient's results to the correct provider, etc. The sum of all three phases is knows as the Total Testing Process (TTP). The QA plan should be set up to measure preanalytic, analytic, and postanalytic quality.

I like to measure test turn around time, calling of critical values, crossmatch:transfusion ratio, blood culture contamination rate, and complaints received. Generally the collection and evaluation of the data is done monthly.

For some QA indicators it is not likely that any lab will ever achieve perfection. For example no lab will ever maintain 0% blood culture contamination rates for long. In this circumstance, you are looking for improvement over time, or at least maintaining the rate in an acceptable range (preferably less than 3% and definitely less than 5% blood culture contamination rate).

If any QA indicator is in the acceptable range, but is slowly deteriorating within the acceptable range, it is best to be proactive. Take action before the numbers deteriorate into the unacceptable range.

Most hospitals have a monthly, quarterly, and annual QA form to fill out. One form is used for each QA indicator for each time period under evaluation (monthly, quarterly or annual). Lab typically uses the hospital-wide forms and does not have its own separate forms for QA.

Let's say that you calculate the blood culture contamination rate and find that it is 6%. This is in the unacceptable range. The data is presented at the relevant committee meetings (Infection Control Committee, Quality Management Committee, etc).

The corrective actions to take include educating the phlebotomists who draw the blood cultures on aseptic technique for drawing. Have the most senior phlebotomist or the Lab Supervisor watch the more junior phlebotomists to make sure they really are swabbing the alcohol or iodine for 30 seconds and allowing it to air dry. The 30 seconds and air dry rules tends to be shortcut, as the phlebotomists are usually in a hurry.

The Lab cannot carry out corrective actions on the nurses without the approval of the nursing administration. If the nurses draw blood cultures, the Lab should inform the Director of Nursing that there is a problem, and ask him or her to address the issue. Usually, the information (high blood culture contamination rate, how to draw a blood culture, etc.) is passed down from the Director of Nursing, to the departmental nursing heads to the individual nurses. Alternatively, the nurses can have one big educational meeting where this information is presented to everybody at once, usually with the infection control nurse present at this meeting as well.

Continue doing this and check how the next month's blood culture contamination rate comes out. If it is improved, and in the acceptable range, you can stop. If it is still not in the acceptable range, you have to keep working on improving it. You will need to continue with the education of the drawing staff. You can add on a policy of collecting a waste red top tube prior to collecting the blood culture bottles.

Continue doing this and see how subsequent months' blood culture contamination rates come out. If it is improved, and in the acceptable range, you can stop. If it is still not in the acceptable range, you have to keep working on it. You can track the contaminated blood cultures back to who drew them. If there is one or a few people that drew most of the contaminated blood cultures, they are singled out for more intensive education and scrutiny on their technique for drawing.

If the employees having problems drawing blood cultures improve their technique, and the contamination rate drops into the acceptable range, you can stop. If these employees do not improve their technique, and still have an unacceptably high contamination rate, they should be sidelined from further drawing of blood cultures.

Eventually, the problem will be fixed, and the blood culture contamination rate will come back into the acceptable range. You may upset many people while trying to fix the problem, and that may be unavoidable. The alternative is sticking your head in the sand and ignoring the problem, which is even worse. Once the problem is fixed, the blood culture contamination rate goes from active intervention to watching the numbers every month. If the problem recurs, repeat the corrective action steps given above.

The information on your efforts to fix the problem, your results and the relevant QA forms are presented on a monthly basis to the relevant committees with quarterly and annual summaries. Document the improvements made, opportunities for further improvement, constraints to improvement and how you have or will overcome the constraints to improvement. The paperwork is filed in the relevant file folders. The same is done for each and every QA indicator that you have picked from the above list.

Let's say that we picked crossmatch:transfusion ratio as a QA indicator, and set a target of no more than 1.5 ratio of crossmatches to transfusions. Here is an example of what the crossmatch:transfusion data will look like after it is compiled:

Blood Utilization Review Committee

DATA COLLECTION for October 2013

Ward	ER	Peds	NICU	Hemo	ICU	Med	OB	L&D	OR
PRBC units crossmatched	50	31	11	0	2	13	7	3	5
PRBC units transfused	45	28	9	0	1	11	5	2	4
Ratio	1.11	1.18	1.22	N/A	2.0	1.18	1.40	1.50	1.25

	Hospital wide total
PRBC units crossmatched	122
PRBC units transfused	105
Ratio	1.16

After compiling the data you then review it. In the above example, the hospital wide crossmatch transfusion ratio is quite good. You want it to be less than 1.5 and it came in much better than this. The ICU falls out with a ratio of 2.0. However with only one unit transfused the ratio for ICU is not really meaningful.

The data is presented at the relevant committee meetings (Blood Utilization Review Committee, Quality Management Committee, etc). If there are no significant fall-outs the data is then filed in the relevant file folder.

If you have a significant fall-out, for example the hospital wide crossmatch:transfusion ratio comes out higher than the 1.5 target you must try to correct the situation. For crossmatch:transfusion ratio this would entail informing the providers that they should only order crossmatches if they are relatively certain that the patient will need transfusion within the next 72 hours.

Next month check to see if this QA indicator has improved. If it is improved, and in the acceptable range, you can stop. If it is still not in the acceptable range, you have to keep working on improving it. Continue educating the providers. If this doesn't improve things, you can have the BUTR committee send letters to offending providers, refer egregious cases to the various departments of the hospital for peer review, etc.

If you persist eventually you will fix the problem. You may upset many people while trying to fix the problem, and that may be unavoidable. The alternative is sticking your head in the sand and ignoring the problem, which is even worse.

The information on your efforts to fix the problem, your results and the relevant QA forms are presented on a monthly basis to the relevant committees with quarterly and annual summaries. Document the improvements made, opportunities for further improvement, constraints to improvement and how you have or will overcome the constraints to improvement. The paperwork is filed in the relevant file folders.

You should keep measuring the same QA indicator (in this example crossmatch:transfusion ratio) on a monthly basis to make sure the problem does not recur. If the problem recurs, repeat the corrective action steps given above.

The same is done for each and every QA indicator that you have picked from the above list. Choose your QA indicators carefully, or you will be working very hard.

You are allowed to change your QA indicators over time. If some of the QA indicators you are watching come out good month after month for an extended period, it may not be worthwhile to continue measuring these QA indicators. The assumption is that your hospital doesn't have a problem in these areas and won't ever have a problem in these areas. If you drop one QA indicator, it is best to add a different QA indicator, or the inspector may think you are slacking off.

The lab Quality Assurance program typically includes complaints and incident reports involving lab. As Lab Director, you will spend a significant portion of your time answering complaints. A complaint is typically defined as an allegation that lab has not followed its own policies and procedures. I define a complaint even more broadly as any customer dissatisfaction with lab.

For example a doctor comes to me complaining that a routine lab test ordered at 3PM was not ready by 4:30PM. I inform that doctor that lab policies allow 24 hours for a routine test to be completed. If you need faster turn around time, order the test as a STAT so as to have results within one hour. To me this counts as a complaint, even though the lab followed its own policies and procedures.

Most complaints are petty, such as the example above. As a Lab Director you will spend a good amount of your time answering to clinicians upset about everything imaginable. In my experience this includes the computer screen is too small to read, the lab did not FAX the results I wanted, I want the lab to print out the test results and courier the printout to my clinic, etc. As you can see there is quite a bit of overlap between complaints and unreasonable clinician demands on lab. I will discuss unreasonable clinician demands on lab at greater length in a later chapter.

More significant complaints are less common and typically involve a clinician's suspicion that there is something wrong with one or more test. An ER doctor has 10 consecutive patients with low platelets and calls you to ask if there is a problem with the platelet testing. A call of this nature should send you into the hematology section immediately. Look at the controls for that day and the prior days of the same month. Did the controls come in on the first try? When was the last calibration? Was the lot changed recently? Does the lot number on the control bottles match the lot number the analyzer is programmed with? Are all the reagents in date with no expired reagents?

Once you are satisfied that there are no problems with the testing, you can call back the doctor in question and reassure that doctor there was no problem with the testing. In this example you'd be calling back the ER doctor and telling him or her that there was no problem with the platelet testing, and yes there really were 10 consecutive patients with low platelets.

The next type of significant clinician complaint involves a problem with one patient's testing. In this scenario the clinician calls and tells you "Patient X has secondary polycythemia, but today's CBC shows severe anemia. Please double-check the results". In this case, when there is only one patient result in question, you have to rule out a switched specimen, or some other type of misdrawing whereby the wrong patient's results are being assigned to the patient in question.

In my experience clinician calls asking "is there a problem with with this one patient's test?" are a false alarm more than 90% of the time. However, you are obligated to follow up on these calls as urgently as possible. If your lab ever does release erroneous results this is the first and most likely way it will get caught. Thus every complaint of this nature is taken seriously and followed up with urgency.

Incident reports are a little different than a complaint. An incident report is an internal hospital document that records information relating to an accident or other unwanted event at the facility. An incident report is filled out by hospital staff whereas a complaint is typically made by a lab customer. Incident reports tend to be of a more serious nature than a complaint. There is some overlap, as it is possible for a complaint to be written up as an incident report.

The most serious incidents I have seen involve switching one patent's specimen and/or lab results with another patient. This typically occurs at the time of drawing with the wrong barcode label put on the wrong tube. This is typically caught when a "delta check" shows wide swings in the patient's results for certain analytes since the prior testing. Delta check is the mandatory comparison of current lab results with any immediate prior lab results to make sure that the current results are consistent with the prior results. I have also seen switched specimens caught when the patient is typed and found to have a different ABO type than what the Blood Bank records indicate.

In my experience if a switch occurs, it is usually caught before the results go out from lab. If switched patient test results get released, you will likely get a call from one or both clinicians involved that today's lab test results for a patient do not fit the clinical picture.

Pull out the tube of blood used for the testing and check the label against the patient identifying information in the computer. The phlebotomists are required to initial all labels on the tubes they draw. Talk to the phlebotomist who drew this specimen and ask if it is possible there was a switch. Check the other test results on that run, to see if some other patient has an unexpected test result that would fit better for the patient in question. If so, this would be evidence of a switch.

If you are trying to rule out a misdraw or switch, you can type the tubes of blood for ABO and Rh, minor blood group antigens, etc. A change in ABO, Rh or minor blood group antigens confirms a specimen misdraw or switch. Unchanged ABO, Rh and minor blood group antigens indicates a switch or misdraw is less likely, but does not completely exclude this. Have the patient in question redrawn and compare the redraw results to the results in question.

The phlebotomist who drew the switched specimens should have immediate corrective action. For such a severe incident, this counseling is done in a closed-door meeting usually by the Lab Supervisor with the section supervisor and Lab Director present in the room. Be as nice as possible. The Lab Supervisor will inform the phlebotomist involved that a switched specimen has been identified and that phlebotomist drew the switched specimen. The phlebotomist involved will usually be very apologetic. The phlebotomist will be informed of the requirement for two patient identifiers before drawing and that switched specimens have the potential to be life-threatening to the patients involved. Further occurrences are considered unacceptable.

Another less common error is testing the right patient, but using the specimen from the wrong time of collection. Let's say I'm in the ICU getting heparinized. My 3AM INR is 1.2 and I am drawn again at 3PM. The 3PM specimen has an INR of 2.5 due to heparinization. The 3PM specimen is drawn and put on a refrigerator rack next to my 3AM specimen. My 3AM specimen is pulled out of the refrigerator inadvertently and run in place of my 3PM specimen. The incorrect result of 1.2 INR is given, and I get a whole lot more heparin than I really need. Later the mistake is caught and the 3PM results are corrected to a 2.5 INR. This sort of mistake indicates carelessness and/or inattention and should prompt immediate corrective action as described for the phlebotomist above.

Any public disturbance in the hospital will generate an incident report. At one hospital I worked at, there were several incident reports involving the Morgue. On several occasions, the family of a deceased patient had a reaction interpreted by the hospital staff as a public disturbance. These were duly written up.

Incident reports are used to document a wide variety of problems, from computer outages to power outages to analyzer breakdowns. If an unexpected event stops the lab or part of the lab from doing testing, it probably needs an incident report. I have seen incident reports generated by earthquakes and hurricanes.

The lab must report to OSHA all accidents, spills, chemical exposures, injuries and biologic exposures. An incident report should be generated for any untoward event in these categories, so as to be able to keep track of any occurrences.

As Lab Director all incident reports involving lab should come across your desk. The incident report form typically has fields to be filled out for investigation, Root Cause Analysis (RCA) and plan of correction to prevent recurrence. You can do the investigation, RCA and plan of correction yourself or more likely delegate this off to the Lab Supervisor.

As the name implies, an RCA tries to identify the root cause of the incident. In one of the examples above the root cause of the problem was that the phlebotomist drew the wrong patient. In order to do an RCA properly you must examine the entire system involved. Why did the phlebotomist draw the wrong patient? Is there a policy in place mandating the phlebotomist to use two patient identifiers? Is there a policy in place requiring all patients to have a hospital wristband in order to be drawn? Is there a policy in place requiring the phlebotomist to label each tube of blood before leaving the patient's room? Can the delta check process be improved so as to be more likely to catch a switched specimen before the results are released from lab?

In order to do an RCA correctly, you must examine the entire process of drawing: The patient comes in to the hospital and has the wristband put on. The patient should be instructed to never alter or remove this wristband. The doctor orders the test in the hospital computer system. The request prints in the phlebotomy printer. The phlebotomist arrives at work and collects up the list of patients to draw. The phlebotomist goes to that patient's room, draws the patient, and somehow gets the wrong barcode label on that tube of blood. The process repeats at the next patient's room. Alternatively, the phlebotomist may have drawn two patients, and applied the barcode labels after the fact. The lab does the testing not realizing that the wrong patient's blood is being used for the testing.

When doing an RCA it is not sufficient to take the easy way out and say "it's all the phlebotomist's fault". This would not be considered an adequate RCA. If your CMS inspector caught you doing this, you'd be cited in the inspection, in effect being told by the inspector to do it the right way.

Another technique for doing an RCA involves repeatedly asking "Why?" until one comes to the root cause of the problem. This technique is mentioned in the COLA literature. In my experience, there is no way to know when you have reached the root cause and it is time to stop asking "Why?". Instead, one could ask "Why?" forever. I prefer the systematic approach given above. It has a defined start, systematic way of looking at the problem, and a defined end point.

After making the RCA you then make a plan of correction to prevent recurrence. For the above example of switched specimens, the plan of correction is to counsel the phlebotomist that made the switch, monitor that phlebotomist's performance closely, and remind all phlebotomists to check two identifiers on all patient's wristbands and label all tubes before leaving the patient's room.

Write the RCA and plan of correction into the appropriate fields of the incident report form. Sign off on the incident report form, and forward it to the next person in line to receive it, typically the hospital Risk Manager or hospital-wide Quality Assurance Coordinator.

In most hospitals it is forbidden to make copies of an incident report form. The completed forms for lab incident reports are usually not stored in lab but instead are stored in the hospital Risk Manager's Office.

Chapter 13 – How to deal with personnel problems

The reason I went into Pathology and Lab Medicine is because it tends to be relatively sheltered from interaction with others. As a Lab Director you will never see a patient directly and never have to tell anyone horribly bad news such as "You have cancer", "You have 3 months left to live", etc.

The Lab Supervisor is tasked with enforcing the rules and regulations on the lab staff including all disciplinary matters. As such the Lab Supervisor will have much more contact with a problem employee than you will. However, as Lab Director one still has to interact with the various personalities found in the typical hospital lab.

In most of the labs I am familiar with the lab staff works together like family. The most frequent problem is the late to work or lazy employee not getting the job done in the time allotted. Significant arguments between 2 employees is rare.

Potentially homicidal or suicidal employees are so rare that I have only seen one each in my 23 years in Pathology and Lab Medicine. It is imperative to spot a potentially homicidal or suicidal employee. The consequences of missing warning signs could be devastating. I will cover these two topics first.

    A. How to spot a potentially homicidal employee

Workplace violence typically involves an adult acting alone. There are typically a series of warning signs given off prior to the event:

1. Male gender. This is really the strongest risk factor. Workplace violence perpetrated by a

    female is virtually unheard of.
 2. The offender is typically a socially withdrawn loner with no friends and no interest in making friends
 3. Gun ownership. Fascination with guns and war. Tends to stockpile ammunition.
 4. Prior history of violence. Prior history of incarceration.
 5. Psychiatric history, especially the types of personality disorder that cause the sufferer to dehumanize others.
 6. History of drug and/or alcohol abuse.
 7. Indirect threats are more likely than direct threats in the run-up to workplace violence.
 8. Triggering event, such as loss of the job, divorce, etc.

My assessment: I would recommend against knowingly hiring any employee with a prior history of violence. If any employee has 3 or more of these risk factors, I will refer them to counseling and specifically ask the counselor to evaluate the employee for potential workplace violence.

In my 23 years in Pathology and Lab Medicine only once have I had contact with a potentially homicidal employee. His name is Fred. I will not mention his last name. He moved from Las Vegas in the late 1990s and took jobs in two different labs in my community. His day job was a full time position in the lab where I worked, which I will refer to as "my lab" for the purpose of this story, even though I don't own this lab. His other job was a part time night job at an outside lab I will refer to as the "other lab" for the purpose of this story.

Fred's performance at my lab was perfectly acceptable. A few people in my lab though he was a little strange, but most people liked him. He didn't seem to be having any major problems. He got good evaluations from the Lab Supervisor at my lab, and got a few routine salary increments over the course of the next few years.

However, Fred was having major problems at the outside lab. The Lab Supervisor at the outside lab had a reputation for being excessively tough, and excessively writing up the subordinate lab staff. Fred got into an escalating series of arguments with this Lab Supervisor sometime around the year 2000. The more Fred argued with this Lab Supervisor, the more this Lab Supervisor wrote Fred up.

This escalating series of arguments and write-ups ended with Fred shouting at the Lab manager "I am going to go home and get my gun. I'll be back" and then storming out of the outside lab. The Lab Supervisor called the police. The police came to the outside lab, took down the complaint, went to Fred's house and arrested Fred.

No one at my lab was aware of what was going on at the outside lab. The way we found out is that Fred didn't show up for work at my lab as scheduled. The lab staff of my lab called Fred's house to see why he no-showed work. The staff were shocked then they found out Fred was in jail because of his confrontation with the Lab Supervisor at the outside lab.

When we found out about this, my lab quietly dropped Fred from the employee rolls. The Personnel Office presumably send a letter to his address telling him he was no longer an employee. He was in jail at the time so likely didn't get the letter. We never heard from Fred again, and this was probably for the best.

I got some follow up from an acquaintance that works at the outside lab. Fred spent about a month in jail waiting for his case to come in front of the Judge. When he came in front of the Judge, the Judge ordered a 30 day psychiatric evaluation. After the 30 day psychiatric evaluation was done the Judge heard the case again. The Psychiatrist said that Fred was not a threat to the outside lab or its Lab Supervisor. The Judge released Fred based on time served, and made a restraining order that Fred is not allowed to come within 500 feet of the outside lab or the outside Lab Supervisor.

Fred moved back to Las Vegas shortly after being released from jail. I had no further contact with him nor did anyone else from my lab.

B. How to spot a potentially suicidal employee

The following are warning signs of a potentially suicidal employee:

1. Adverse or traumatic life event, especially divorce or death of a spouse
2. Mental illness, especially major depression. The clinical manifestations of depression include deep sadness, loss of interest in things one used to care about, making comments about being hopeless, helpless, or worthless, trouble sleeping and eating, sudden weight gain or loss.
3. History of alcohol and/or substance abuse.
4. Talking or writing about death or suicide.
5. One or more prior suicide attempts.
6. Family history of mental disorder or substance abuse
7. Gun ownership, with gun kept in the home.
8. Chronic physical illness, including chronic pain
9. Gender is not a risk factor. Suicides occur at about equal rates in both genders.

My assessment: If any employee has 2 or more of these risk factors, I will refer them to counseling and specifically ask the counselor to evaluate the employee for potential suicide.

In my 23 years in Pathology and Lab Medicine only once have I had contact with an employee I thought was potentially suicidal. In September, 2013 I was acting as an off-site Lab Director for a small hospital lab. I was remote from the Lab and communicating by E-mail. In mid-September the Lab Supervisor E-mailed me that an employee showed up late for a scheduled 3 to 11 PM shift arriving approximately 4:30PM. According to the Lab Supervisor, she is going through a divorce and has to pick up her children from school and can't make it in to work until after 4PM.

On September 12, 2013 from me to the Lab Supervisor: I think the best way to handle this is to sit down with her, and try to work out a schedule that will accommodate her without unduly inconveniencing lab. If she has to pick the children up from school at 4PM, and there is no one else that can pick her children up from school, then we should try to arrange things so that she starts work at 5PM. Ask the day shift if there is anyone willing to work an extra two hours every day at the end of their shift, to cover the 3PM to 5PM block.

On September 18 from the Lab Supervisor to me: She came to me in tears the other day. In labs were no one wanted to work odd shifts, holidays, etc a monthly rotational schedule was implemented.

On September 19 from me to the Lab Supervisor: I do not know her personally. Where I work, there is counseling on site for employees having personal problems. If an employee was having the same problems as her (getting divorced, repeatedly late for work, crying at work, etc.) that employee would get mandatory referral to the internal counselor. She is sending out a lot of red flags that she is having personal problems and may need help. If you have an internal counseling service, please refer her.

C. How to deal with 2 lab employees that do not get along

Minor disagreements between two employees can usually be resolved by the next person up the chain of command. Usually it is a negotiating process whereby the supervisor offers one person something of value (e.g. overtime) in exchange for doing something the tech otherwise wouldn't want to do (e.g. work in a different section of Lab).

The situation whereby two people in lab truly hate each other is uncommon in my experience. However, when it happens you will never forget it.

I graduated from training in 1996 and went to work in a hospital where two Blood Bank techs had been having a long-running argument. I was hired into the Pathologist position at that hospital. The Lab Director at that hospital was older, nearing retirement, and tired of constantly having to referee the arguments between these two Blood Bank techs.

The Lab Director had long since given up on getting these two quarreling techs to agree on anything. When I started work there, he immediately delegated me Blood Bank. This meant that he could distance himself from the two quarreling techs and I would have to deal directly with them.

When I started work at that hospital the Blood Bank was divided into donor side and transfusion side. One of the Blood Bank techs was on the transfusion side and the other was on the donor side. Each of them kept accusing the other of making more work for the other.

It was my assignment to try to get these two techs to bury the hatchet. First, I spoke to them individually. The tech working the donor side of Blood Bank said that the tech working in transfusion side is making more work for the donor side of Blood Bank. The tech working the transfusion side of Blood bank said that the tech working in donor side is making more work for the transfusion side of Blood Bank.

While meeting individually with the techs I explained to each of them that yes, transfusion side makes more work for donor side, and yes, donor side makes more work for transfusion side, but if both sides stop working, the Blood Bank as a whole would stop working.

This did not help. The next approach that I tried is called "one big meeting". In this approach, the two quarreling techs are called into a meeting along with their respective supervisors, the Lab Supervisor, and the Lab Director. I called everyone in for one big meeting. In this meeting the supervisory people tried to negotiate away all the problems, and tried to cajole and coerce the two quarreling techs to stop arguing so much.

This approach of having one big meeting is popular in the management literature. In my experience it does not work. The techs may pretend to get along for the course of the meeting.

However, as soon as the meeting is over they will go back to arguing. That is exactly what happened. In this case the two techs were back to arguing within one week of the one big meeting.

I proposed merging the donor side and transfusion side of Blood Bank, so that it would not appear that one side was making more work for the other. This was not possible due to the different credentials of the people working on the different sides of Blood Bank.

I proposed hiring techs for Blood Bank or reshuffling techs from the main part of the lab into Blood Bank so as to spread the workload around. The Lab Supervisor felt there wasn't enough work to justify more techs in Blood Bank and the two quarreling techs in Blood Bank did not have excessive workload. In other words, the Lab Supervisor felt that the quarreling Blood Bank techs were not justified in their complaints about their workload, each making more work for the other, etc.

The next thing to try is to separate the two arguing techs in time and space as much as is possible. If one tech can "float" send that tech to a different section in lab such that there is minimal contact with the other tech. Reassign one or both of the techs to the swing shift and/or graveyard shift such that the only time they see each other is at change of shift.

In reality what happened is that these two techs continued their arguing throughout the remainder of the 1990s. It did not end until the donor side tech moved to a job in a different part of the same hospital around the year 2000.

In my career of 23 years in Pathology and Lab Medicine I have not seen lab techs argue so much before or after this episode. Thankfully this was an isolated episode.

D. How to deal with a disagreement between employees inside and outside lab

In this permutation, the disagreement is between one or more lab staff and one or more employee that works in a different part of the same hospital. This is relatively common and I could give multiple examples. In order to keep this chapter brief I will only give one example.

One of the hospitals I have worked at was a small community hospital with only one doctor staffing the ER at night. This one doctor was older, but very energetic. The ER had a heavy volume. Most nights there were fairly large number of patients coming in, but a lot of the work was routine. In this small community the clinics all closed at 6PM. All the minor cough, cold and flu cases came to the ER after 6PM and the ER was loaded with routine work.

This doctor insisted on having a phlebotomist by her side the entire night so that as this doctor went from patient to patient the doctor could order lab tests and have them drawn on the spot. The lab policy allows the phlebotomists to take a 30 minute meal break at the midpoint of the 8 hour shift as long as there is no STAT work to be done. This ER doctor would object to the 30 minute meal break. This ER doctor wanted a phlebotomist by her side the entire 8 hours she was working.

There is only one phlebotomist scheduled on the night shift, and the night duty would rotate among a pool of 5 phlebotomists. Most of the phlebotomists did as told, skipping their 30 minute meal break and working 8 hours straight to keep this ER doctor happy. One phlebotomist objected. This resulted in a mutual write-up whereby the ER doctor wrote up the phlebotomist for "attitude" and the phlebotomist wrote up the ER doctor for "attitude".

As a Lab Director, all write-ups and incident reports related to lab should come across your desk. If it is important you will usually be informed at the start of the next working day. The mutual write-up between the ER doctor and the phlebotomist was seen as relatively unimportant; the paperwork came across my desk with other routine paperwork well after the fact.

I dutifully carried out my part. I talked with the phlebotomist and asked her side of the story. She is diabetic and needs to eat at regular intervals. The ER doctor gave the phlebotomist "attitude" when the phlebotomist said that she had to take off for a 30 minute meal and that the routine testing can wait.

The ER doctor works the night shift, and I did not speak directly to the ER doctor. I left a message for the ER doctor to call me during the daytime hours regarding the phlebotomy coverage of ER. The message was left for me that the ER doctor considers it essential to have a phlebotomist present the entire time, with no breaks.

Let's think this through. The lab policy says that the phlebotomist gets a 30 minute meal if there are no STATs to be drawn. The routine work can wait 30 minutes. I have never heard of any other ER doctor needing to have a phlebotomist right by their side the entire shift. At this point, I make the judgment call that the ER doctor is being unreasonable.

As Lab Director your authority begins and ends with lab. You can rearrange the phlebotomist schedule such that the diabetic phlebotomist only works the day shift, and the other phlebotomists work the night shift with the ER doctor in question.

As Lab Director, you do not have authority over an ER doctor. The chain of command is such that the ER doctor answers to the ER department head who in turn answers to the hospital Medical Director.

The best thing to do at this point is to call the ER department head and inform the ER department head that there has been a mutual write up between the ER doctor and a phlebotomist. The lab thinks that the ER doctor is being unreasonable. Even so, the lab will schedule a different phlebotomist at night so hopefully this will not recur. The Lab considers the case to be closed, unless and until there are further write-ups between this ER doctor and the phlebotomists.

In general for a situation such as this it is important to resolve the disagreement as quickly as possible. If you leave the same phlebotomist working with the same ER doctor, the result is likely to be intractable arguments and a firestorm of write-ups. From an administrative perspective, a firestorm of write-ups between two employees is very difficult to deal with, a real headache. It is best to separate the two before the situation comes to this.

The switching of the phlebotomists solved the lab's problem with this ER doctor. The other phlebotomists did not mind working 8 hours straight.

Let's suppose the same ER doctor and the other phlebotomists start doing mutual write-ups. In this situation the best approach is to call a meeting with the ER department head and the ER doctor in question. Talk to the ER department head in advance of this meeting and make sure the ER department head will back you in this meeting. In the meeting explain to the ER doctor in question that the phlebotomist really is allowed to take a 30 minute meal break if there are no STATs to be drawn. Ask the ER to accommodate this by assigning a nurse or other ER staff to do the phlebotomy for the 30 minutes the phlebotomist is on break.

E. How to deal with the chronically late to work employee

Work ethic is not distributed evenly among mankind. I am relatively hardworking, putting in an average of 10 hour days five days a week. That is slightly more than the typical Pathologist/Lab Director, but not as hardworking as a surgeon.

At the other end of the spectrum are people who consider 6 or 7 hours of work a day and/or three day weekends to be the normal and natural state of affairs. I have no problem with this as long as it is acknowledged that the person is working part-time by the definition the lab uses. Full time is defined as 40 or more hours per week, part time is anything less.

If a person shows up late to work in Lab it creates a problem for the other people working in Lab. The Lab staff schedule typically has to be rearranged at the last minute with someone on the prior shift asked to keep working until the late employee shows up. I will refer to this late arriving employee as CLTW for Chronically Late To Work. In my experience the CLTW employee is the most common problem employee in Lab.

When an employee in lab is CLTW it can be very demoralizing to the other lab staff. A lab tech or phlebotomist has to stay late every time the CLTW employee arrives late. The other lab techs and phlebotomists have family, children to pick up from school, etc. If the situation is not corrected the other lab staff will eventually come to believe that they should not have to work hard if the CLTW employee does not have to work hard. Once an employee becomes CLTW they will not usually start showing up on time until they receive one or more corrective actions. In this circumstance, the corrective action reassures the other lab staff that something is being done to fix the problem.

The Lab Supervisor is generally the person tasked with scheduling of lab techs. The CLTW employee can be a big headache for the Lab Supervisor, but is usually not a big problem for the Lab Director.

As a Lab Director you will only see the CLTW employee if the Lab Supervisor and/or section supervisor have been doing multiple write-ups on the CLTW employee. In my experience this is uncommon and the CLTW employee will show up on time to work after the first write-up or two.

Motivating the CLTW employee to work hard is another story. This falls first on the section supervisor. If the section supervisor fails it then falls on the Lab Supervisor. You will only see the CLTW tech if the section supervisor and/or Lab Supervisor have been doing multiple write-ups on that tech.

In my 23 years in Pathology and Lab Medicine there have been only one or two instances where this came across my desk in the form of multiple write-ups that I had to sign off on. In these cases, I asked the CLTW tech to get a medical evaluation to make sure there was no correctable condition (hypothyroidism, anemia, diabetes, etc.) that was curtailing their ability to work hard. I did not document this request in writing.

If the tech refused medical evaluation or if the medical evaluation came back with nothing wrong, I would sign off on the write-ups and forward them to the Personnel Office. The Lab Supervisor and the Personnel Office would do the dirty work of removing the CLTW tech, or renegotiating the CLTW tech's position as a part-time position.

Another variation of this occurs when a lab tech chronically abuses leave time. In one of the labs I worked at, there was a lab tech named John who liked to take annual leave the entire week between Christmas and New Year. Any year that he did not get scheduled for this leave, he would call in sick the entire week.

The problem is that everyone else also wants time off at Christmas. The scheduling of leave is on a first-come, first-served basis. At this particular lab, the annual leave scheduling calendar opens in January. I encouraged John to put in his Christmas leave request 11 months in advance, when the annual leave calendar opens, so that he could get his wish of leave time at Christmas.

One year John lost this race to other techs, who put in their request for Christmas leave first. When Christmas time came, John called in sick the 4 working days between Christmas and New Year's Day. The hospital's policy on leave time requires a doctor's sick excuse when sick leave time is used for 3 or more consecutive working days. John was asked to produce his doctor's excuse but he could not produce one. The hospital's administrative manual will tell you what to do in this circumstance. In this particular lab, if the tech cannot produce a doctor's excuse the tech is assigned leave without pay for the days missed.

A lab tech who does this once a year is not a major problem. Any lab tech doing this frequently will quickly become a problem. In most labs the Lab Supervisor is tasked with all lab tech scheduling issues to include employees who abuse leave time. As Lab Director, all you have to do is sign off on the write-ups done by the Lab Supervisor and/or section supervisor.

Chapter 14 – Physician and administrator demands on lab and physician ordering practices

This is really the most onerous part about being a Lab Director. Most hospital administrators see lab as a cost center and are constantly looking to cut costs. Most physicians expect to have unlimited access to lab testing. As Lab Director, you are caught between a rock and a hard place.

As Lab Director, you don't have enough time to police every test ordered by every physician. Thus the most expensive and most esoteric tests are the ones that come under the most scrutiny Even so most doctors are upset when I call to ask the indications for doing this testing, or question the need for any given test. If the doctor says that it is a medical necessity, I generally allow the testing.

I have seen many instances whereby doctors made unreasonable demands on lab. In one such instance, a hematologist/oncologist wanted to do bone marrow exams during the nighttime hours. In this episode, the hematologist/oncologist was at her clinic during the 8AM to 5PM time frame, went home, ate dinner then came in to the hospital between 7PM to 9PM to do rounds. If any patient needed a bone marrow, she wanted to do it at that time.

The problem with this is that the lab's day shift is long gone by 7PM and the swing shift is a skeleton crew. There were only 3 or 4 people on swing shift, and none off them could be spared to assist with the bone marrow exam. Part of the bone marrow testing was sent out, and the reference lab would not send a courier after 5PM. The specimen would wait for pickup until the next working day.

This hematologist/oncologist was insistent that lab had to accommodate her schedule, and not the other way around. We came to an agreement that the hematologist/oncologist would have to schedule all nighttime bone marrows well in advance so that lab could arrange for an additional person on swing shift. The reference lab agreed to send the courier up to 9PM if we scheduled this in advance.

Hospital Administrator demands on lab almost always come in the form of a generic "cut costs". The labs that I have worked at have no fat left to cut. Cutting costs means cutting services.

When I get called into an administrator's office and told to cut costs, my response is that the only way to cut costs is to cut services. I mention a few things that can be done to save money - close the lab at night, curtail blood bank services, etc. I ask the administrator to pick which one of these to cut. Since cutting any of these would be onerous, and would result in a backlash from the medical staff, the administrator usually backs off at this point.

In the rare instance whereby the administrator wants to cut services, I make sure that the medical staff knows where the decision came from. This way the backlash will be against the administrator and not me.

Chapter 15 – Professional relations. Making sure you are not a problem employee

As an employee, the number of possible rule violations is virtually limitless. The Code of Federal Regulations is tens of thousands of pages. Most municipalities have thousands of pages of municipal codes. Most hospital's administrative manual is in the hundreds of pages. I couldn't repeat it all here, to tell you what not to do, or I would end up writing the longest book in history.

However, some basic rules are universal. Obey the laws of the community in which you live. Do not make unwanted advances to another employee in your workplace. Do not discriminate. Do not use vulgar language or dirty words in your workplace. Avoid conflicts of interest. Avoid even the appearance of a conflict of interest. Do not divulge confidential information. In other words, respect the basic rights of everyone around you.

As a Lab Director you will be supervisory to a part of a hospital where maybe 20 to 50 people work. You should try to set a good example for those below you. Lead by example.

    A. What to wear to work

Most hospitals have a dress code that is very vague. The following is a quote of one hospital's entire dress code: "Dress in a neat, clean, professionally appropriate manner". This is so vague as to be useless.

In most hospitals the personnel who will come into contact with patients are held to a higher dress standard than the personnel that will not have patient contact. As a Lab Director, you will not have patient contact on most working days. However, you will be enforcing dress code on the lab staff that does have patient contact. In my opinion, you should be dressed at least as well as the people you are enforcing dress code on; or else your enforcement of the dress code will be seen as hypocrisy

In my 23 years in Pathology and Lab Medicine I have worked in widely disparate geographic locations. The dress code varies by locale. The description given below should be appropriate for most of the continental US.

For men: Wear dress pants, typically a dark color, without patterns. Wear a lighter colored dress shirt, long sleeve is preferred but short sleeve is acceptable. The shirt should be ironed or pressed. Wear a tie and a jacket or sport coat. The jacket or sport coat should be the exact same color as the pants. Wear dress shoes, typically dark color. This combination of clothes is known as a "business suit".

For women: Skirt or trousers, with matching jacket and a blouse. More variation is allowed than for men.

While in the continental US my usual daily routine is to dress up in the business suit in the morning. When I come to work the first thing I do is to take off the sport coat and set it on a hanger in my office area. The business suit minus the sport coat is called "business casual" or something similar. When going out for lunch and at the end of the day, I put the sport coat back on as the last thing I do before heading out of the office.

In some areas, the dress code is more casual. In the time I worked on Guam, some of the attending physicians came into the hospital in jeans and sneakers, and did their rounds wearing jeans and sneakers. There was even a story about a surgeon who was at the beach on the weekend, and was paged to come in for an appendectomy. He came into the hospital wearing nothing but swimming trunks, and had to change into scrubs to see the patient.

As far as I can tell, the dress code for Hawaii and the US Pacific territories is:

For men: Wear khaki colored cotton trousers and a shirt with floral patterns. Wear sneakers or similar casual shoes.

For women: Wear a skirt with floral patterns.

    B. Always know your relationship to your employer

I graduated from training in 1996 and took my first job as an attending Physician. I was hired into a municipal hospital on a GG1 form, a one page form that did not stipulate any conditions other than my salary and that I was full-time. This is what they offered me and I accepted. I was fresh out of training at the time, and did not have experience in negotiating salary, terms, etc.

The same hospital hired a variety of doctors on a variety of different terms. Some were hired as locum tenens, some were hired on contracts, some were hired on GG1 forms. Depending on the nature of the employment, some did or did not get callback pay, some did or did not have to clock in and clock out in the hospital's computer timecard system.

At the start of my employment, I was told that I had to clock in and clock out in the hospital's computer timecard system. I was not told anything about callback time. Over the course of the next 2 years and 9 months, I was called back a few times in the evenings and on weekends. I clocked in and clocked out as a callback. Some callback pay accrued during this time.

In March, 1999 the Medical Director called me in to his office and told me I was not eligible for callback pay. I had accrued about $3800 in callback pay over the course of the prior 2 years and 9 months. My base pay at the time was $156,000 per year so this was less than one percent of my base pay over the course of that time. I apologized to the Medical Director and said that he could make me a bill and I would pay back the $3800 in disputed callback pay.

The Medical Director was disproportionately upset about the callback pay. I found out later that the hospital was starting to have financial problems about this time. The Hospital Administrator had been repeatedly criticizing the Medical Director in private over excessive physician pay. The Medical Director took it out on me, chewing me out over a trivial amount of callback pay.

I made a point of being as nice as possible to the Medical Director. A few weeks later he made a bill for the $3800. I paid the bill the same day, and gave the Medical Director a copy of the canceled check.

Months later, sometime towards the end of 1999, I was offered a contract at the same hospital. I took the contract to my private attorney for review. I spent a long time in the attorney's office talking about the proposed contract, the GG1 form signed in 1996 and the callback pay. The attorney said that the Medical Director was wrong. I really was entitled to the $3800 callback pay. The attorney offered to sue for the disputed $3800. I said that it was best to take no action. The amount in question is trivial, and any action to reclaim the callback pay would only antagonize the hospital administration.

I have told this story to many people. Most people think I should have come out fighting, and given the Medical Director an argument over the $3800. The decision to turn the other cheek or not to turn the other cheek is a personal decision. I can't tell other people what to do in the same circumstance. Neither can anyone else tell me not to turn the other cheek. There are however a few take home points here:

1. Always know your relationship to your employer. In the above story, I did not know in advance if I was or was not entitled to callback pay
2. Never antagonize your employer unless it is absolutely necessary
3. In every situation where you will be negotiating, try to imagine the playing field from the point of view of your counterparty. Imagine that you are the Medical Director and you have just been called on the carpet for excessive physician salary. If you can imagine yourself in the Medical Director's predicament, you will understand why the Medical Director is doing what he does, and you will have some common ground to negotiate.

C. Avoid conflicts of interest

The term "conflict of interest" refers to when an individual or organization is involved in multiple related interests or transactions, one of which could possibly influence the motivation for an act in the other.

The term "arm's length transaction" refers to when the parties in a transaction are independent, equal and unrelated to each other. Any given transaction is either conflicted or arms length (not conflicted).

In 1996 I graduated from training and took my first attending level job at a hospital in a small community. I was hired into the Pathologist position. The Lab Director at that hospital had an outside job working as a the lab director at an outpatient lab. The outpatient lab was a subsidiary of a large reference lab that the hospital had been sending its send-out specimens to.

This relationship was conflicted in two ways. First, the hospital Lab Director could divert work to the outside lab. As in any lab, some tests must obviously be sent out and some tests must be obviously done in-house. However, there are also many classes of specimens that are a "judgment call" as to whether to send out or examine in-house.

The conflict of interest arises from the temptation to send as much work to the outside lab as possible, so as to have less workload (i.e. less work for the same pay) at the hospital lab.

Secondly, the hospital Laboratory Director must determine if the refrence Lab is doing a good job examining specimens from the hospital. The conflict of interest arises from the temptation to look the other way and/or cover up mistakes made by the reference lab.

From what I have been told, this small community had very limited numbers of qualified people in most fields, so the same people tend to occupy multiple different positions of authority at the same time.

There are not enough qualified people in this small community for all transactions to be arm's length (not conflicted). In order to have all the Lab Director positions at arm's length, one person would need to be Lab Director at the hospital, a different person Lab Director at each of multiple outside clinics, a different person Lab Director at Public Health, etc. Since there are not enough qualified people to fill all these positions, the Conflicts of Interest are tolerated as the least bad option.

Eventually, that hospital Lab Director position was reshuffled. The hospital Lab Director retired, but retained his lab directorship at the outside clinic. I took over the hospital Lab Director position when it was vacated by retirement. Thus the conflict of interest was resolved amicably by reshuffling the position.

Later, I would take a position in a different small community. In August 2013 I was hired to "turnaround" a troubled lab in a remote area. The Lab Director had just quit, and the Lab Supervisor had been fired two years prior. When I started work at that lab, my first priory was to get the lab past an upcoming CMS inspection. After passing that CMS inspection, I went through the records to see how the Lab got into its troubled situation in the first place.

There was only one person in that small community who was qualified to be a Lab Supervisor and willing to take the Lab Supervisor position at the hospital. The hospital had a two other ASCP certified lab techs but they were adamant that they would not take the Lab Supervisor position. They did not want the Lab Supervisor position and the hospital regulations would not allow for involuntary promotion.

The only person who was qualified for the Lab Supervisor position and willing to fill the position also had part ownership in an outside lab in the same community.

Again the problem crops up that a small community has very limited numbers of qualified people in most fields. There are not enough qualified people for all transactions to be arm's length (not conflicted).

In this case, the Lab Supervisor cooked up a scheme whereby the paying patients would be diverted from the hospital lab to the private lab he had part ownership of. The non-paying patients coming to his private lab would be diverted to the hospital lab.

This scheme was caught. I do not know exactly how it came to light, but that does not matter for the purpose of this story. This person was immediately forced to resign from the hospital Lab Supervisor position as soon as the scheme was caught. This was a serious blow to the hospital's lab, as there was no replacement for the Lab Supervisor. The hospital administration would not have taken this decision lightly. The lab fell into disarray and later the Lab Director quit. When I took over the leadership role in this lab, I had to carry out both the Lab Director and Lab Supervisor work, as there was no one else available to do it.

The point of this story is to avoid conflicts of interest. Avoid even the appearance of a conflict of interest. There may be situations in which you have to take on two conflicted positions since both positions are necessary and no one else is available to fill them. If you find yourself in this position, never ever act on the conflict of interest. If you act on a conflict of interest you are almost certain to get caught, your punishment will be severe and deservedly so.

Chapter 16 – Lab tech hiring, orientation, competency testing, promotion, retention and discipline

Lab techs can be divided into technicians and technologists. Technicians typically have two years of post-secondary education (i.e. an associate's degree) while technologists have four years of post-secondary education (i.e. a bachelor's degree).

The CLIA requirements for high complexity testing personnel are given in 42 CFR § 493.1489. The requirements for moderate complexity testing personnel are lower. However, in the typical hospital lab there is a mix of waived, moderate and high complexity testing. A tech must be able to go back and forth from one analyzer to another, hence the high complexity testing personnel requirements given in 42 CFR § 493.1489 serve as the minimum hiring criteria for lab techs at every hospital lab I have worked at.

To briefly summarize the 42 CFR § 493.1489 requirements a lab tech must have an associate degree in laboratory science or higher level degree (doctorate, master's, or bachelor's in laboratory science, MD, DO, or DPM) or meet criteria from a list considered equivalent training and/or experience. The tech must be licensed if licensure is required by the State the lab is located in. Anyone grandfathered under older rules can continue to work as a lab tech.

In my 23 years in Pathology and Lab Medicine, I have only once seen CMS inspectors question a lab tech's credentials. This occurred at a small municipal hospital that had hired me to "turnaround" its troubled lab. The lab was under heavy regulatory scrutiny mainly due to reagent outages. A team of CMS inspectors had been dispatched for a re-inspection.

The CMS inspectors completed this re-inspection relatively quickly, and had some spare time on their hands. They went through the personnel files, which I have never seen done at any other CMS inspection. They found that an older tech did not have documentation in his file of his military training as a Medical Laboratory Specialist. This was a 50 week course offered by the US Military prior to April 25, 1995. Without the training certificate in the tech's personnel file, it looked like the lab tech was a high school graduate doing high complexity testing.

The lab tech in question was called in during the inspection to speak with the CMS inspectors. The tech had a copy of this training certificate at home. The tech was sent home to get a copy of his training certificate so as to produce it to the inspectors. The certificate was decades old, and the tech had been working at that same hospital for decades. The personnel file indicated that the tech had produced a copy of this certificate at the time of hiring. The certificate should have been in the personnel file, but it was not there. Somehow a copy of the certificate had been lost in the sands of time from this tech's personnel file.

The tech was able to produce a copy of the training certificate at the time of the inspection. This satisfied the CMS inspectors, they did not issue a citation. Later the tech asked the military to produce a copy directly to the lab. The military had a hard time finding the records for this decades old training, but did eventually produce it, mailing it to the lab.

CLIA makes the Lab Director responsible for adequate staffing of the lab. In my experience, recruitment of lab techs is very difficult, especially in the remote areas I have been working. From talking with others in the field, I think that the US as a whole has a shortage of lab techs. CLIA mandates that you have to hire adequate staffing, but frankly, there aren't enough qualified applicants to fill all of America's lab tech positions.

The best source for hiring lab techs is word of mouth. If you tell enough people in the lab field that your lab is hiring techs, you will eventually receive a call from a lab tech interested in working at your facility. While you are telling everyone else in the lab business that you are hiring for your lab, they will likely tell you that they have vacant positions in their labs that they would like to hire for.

If word of mouth doesn't work. Try putting advertisements in the magazines most often read by lab techs – Advance for Medical Laboratory Professionals, American Journal of Clinical Pathology (AJCP), etc.

I prefer word of mouth for hiring lab techs. When using word of mouth you will mostly get applications from techs that have worked at nearby labs. You will probably know that tech personally or by reputation. When you call to verify the references, you will personally know the Lab Supervisor on the other end of the phone call. I prefer getting the reference from a known quantity; someone I can trust.

An applicant responding to a journal advertisement will likely be from the other end of the country, an unknown quantity. The references will include an unknown Lab Supervisor from across the country. When you call this unknown Lab Supervisor, he or she will most likely only say positive things about the applicant. This Lab Supervisor doesn't know who you are; and likely would not feel comfortable saying anything negative about the applicant. You will have no idea if you can trust the reference.

Recruiting lab techs right out of school is common. One of the municipalities I worked at had a lab tech program at the local University which graduated about 30 students a year. Most years the entire graduating class of 30 lab techs had hiring arrangements in place months before they graduated. The local hospitals would recruit these students during the middle of their fourth year at school. At the time I was working at a municipal hospital which had a slow recruitment process. As a result of slow recruitment, this municipal hospital lost out on the best and brightest students, and had to take whatever students barely passed.

Later the University involved started having financial problems and closed this lab tech program. The University saw it as a small and unimportant program. All the local hospital labs protested the closing of the lab tech program, but the University stood firm saying that they could no longer afford the program. This only served to worsen the lab tech shortage in that municipality.

Recruitment of lab techs is oftentimes a "hard sell" with the hospital administration. The typical hospital administration is very cost-conscious and always looking to cut costs. Salary is one of the biggest expenses in the typical lab. The hospital administration typically wants to keep this to a minimum.

In this situation, the best thing to do is to keep track of the overtime hours and overtime salary paid to the existing lab techs. The overtime is typically paid at time and a half or more. If the overtime amounts to much more than the salary of a tech, you can tell the hospital administration that hiring a new tech would be a cost saving measure which would eliminate much of the overtime.

Most hospital labs I am aware of are short of staff and many are very short. I only know of a few hospital labs that have no vacancies in their lab tech positions. The typical hospital lab gets by with the existing staffing by making heavy use of overtime. If staffing drops further, the next step is to send out as much non-essential testing as possible.

Sending a test to a reference lab is typically much more expensive than doing the same test in-house. When the bill comes back from the reference lab, present the bill to the hospital administration. This usually gets the hospital administration's attention, and they will develop a sense of urgency in the lab tech hiring.

If staffing was to drop further, eventually essential services would need to be curtailed. I have only seen a few instances in which a hospital lab become so short of staff as to curtail essential services. In all instances, the backlash from the medical staff is so severe that the hospital administration quickly becomes motivated to hire lab staff.

There are a variety of certifying agencies for lab techs. The two I am most familiar with are American Society for Clinical Pathology (ASCP) and American Medical Technologists (AMT). CLIA does not recognize any of these certifying agencies. As far as I am concerned any lab tech with US training and an ASCP or AMT certification as a lab technician or lab technologist is good to go. I will not question their underlying education.

If they have work experience I am much more concerned about their recent evaluations than training that may be decades remote. If they are just graduating from training, they will get started out in entry level positions with little responsibility until they can prove themselves

Occasionally you will be faced with evaluating foreign lab tech credentials. I have seen an occasional international applicant with the ASCPi (international ASCP) certification. My understanding is that the holder of ASCPi certification has training in all areas except US regulatory issues.

It would probably be difficult for someone with ASCPi certification to fill the Lab Supervisor position in the US. The Lab Supervisor position deals with regulatory issues, and the ASCPi certification specifically excludes US regulatory issues. There should be no problem with someone holding an ASCPi certification and filling a bench tech or section supervisor position.

CLIA requires an equivalency evaluation for foreign lab tech credentials. The equivalency evaluation has to be performed by a nationally recognized organization or their affiliates. Such organizations include the National Association of Credential Evaluation Services (NACES), the Association of International Credential Evaluators (AICE) and others.

These organizations charge for the evaluation for foreign credentials. In general this cost burden falls on the applicant. In most labs, in order to consider a foreign-trained applicant for a lab tech position the equivalency evaluation must be submitted along with application. Without the equivalency evaluation, it is very hard to compare US and foreign credentials. Thus, the application is not considered complete until the equivalency evaluation is submitted.

In states where lab tech licensure is required, that license is the single most important credential for hiring. The hospitals I have worked at have all been in states that did not require lab tech licensure. In these states when evaluating the credentials of an applicant for a lab tech position, the most important point to look for is certification by one of the lab tech certifying agencies (ASCP, AMT, etc.). An exception to this certification requirement has to be made for students and recent graduates. They will not be able to sit for the certifying exam until about a year after graduation.

Next most important are the references, recent job evaluations, and grades in school. Be wary of any recent graduate that just barely passed, and had to repeat multiple classes in order to graduate. In my experience any hardworking person of average intelligence should be able to get through lab tech school with no problems. The barely passing student is either lacking in intelligence or lacking in effort or both.

The interview has the least importance in my lab. In my experience, a good talker is unlikely to be a hard worker, and vice versa. In the interview style will win out over substance. In my lab, the interview is done to weed out unacceptable candidates. There are a few red flags in the interview that will disqualify a candidate or reduce their ranking.

In the interview you are looking for a lab tech that can think in a linear, logical manner. Ask the applicant how to do typical lab procedures such as phlebotomy or operating an analyzer. Multiple "I don't know" answers disqualifies the applicant. If the applicant is able to answer, but the steps of the procedure are given completely out of order, the applicant's ranking is reduced. If the response is a completely jumbled "word salad" the applicant is disqualified. If the applicant knows the steps of every procedure by heart and recites them all in the correct order, the applicant is moved up in ranking.

In my experience most people can hold themselves together long enough to get through an interview. I am aware of one lab tech passing the interview, and turning out to have a major alcohol problem. This lab tech was only able to stay sober on the day of the interview. At the other end of the spectrum, I have known very bright students who were so shy that they interviewed poorly. They became so intimidated at the interview they began talking in "word salad". Thus in my experience the interview is of little value.

CLIA makes the Lab Director responsible for ensuring that the lab staff are appropriately trained and demonstrate competency prior to testing patient specimens. In virtually every lab I have ever been to, this is delegated to the Lab Supervisor and/or section supervisor.

In my lab, when a lab tech is newly hired, that tech must go through orientation prior to doing any testing. Orientation usually consists of having the tech read the procedure manual for the section of lab they will be assigned to (this should take no more than 2 working days) and then having the section supervisor show the new lab tech the procedures for testing in that area of lab. Then the section supervisor will watch as the new lab tech does some testing. This should take no more than 2 weeks from the time the tech starts. The section supervisor will then sign off on the orientation paperwork, attesting that the newly hired tech is competent in that section of lab.

This stage of competency testing is very basic. I have only seen a few lab techs that needed to repeat orientation. I have never seen a lab tech fail orientation on the second try. If anyone repeatedly fails the orientation, inform the Personnel Office and ask for them to remove the employee.

Under CLIA the following are the minimum requirements for competency testing for all laboratory testing personnel. The competency testing must be done for each person, each test every year. It should evaluate competency to perform test procedures and report test results promptly, accurately and proficiently. The procedures for evaluation of the competency of the staff must include, but are not limited to

1. Direct observations of routine patient test performance, including patient preparation, if applicable, specimen handling, processing and testing
2. Monitoring the recording and reporting of test results
3. Review of intermediate test results or worksheets, quality control records, proficiency testing results, and preventive maintenance records
4. Direct observations of performance of instrument maintenance and function checks
5. Assessment of test performance through testing previously analyzed specimens, internal blind testing samples or external proficiency testing samples
6. Assessment of problem solving skills.

The reference is 42 CFR § 493.1413 (8).

CLIA mandates competency testing at 6 months after hiring and annually thereafter for all lab testing personnel. The competency assessment should evaluate the tech for all phases of testing, preanalytic, analytic and postanalytic. There should be direct observation of skills, not just a written test. I will give an example of a competency assessment document below.

MY LAB		COMPETENCY TESTING FORM	MY PROCEDURE MANUAL
Title	**Section**	**Type of Evaluation**	**Employee Name:**
Training and Competency Checklist	Blood Bank	☐ Initial Training ☐ Annual Competency ☐ Other: _____	Position Title: _____ Date of Hire: _____ Date of Assignment: _____

See Page 2 For Instructions to Complete Form

	Policy, Procedure, Function	Y	N	N/A
	TRANSFUSION SERVICE			
1	Fundamental knowledge of Blood Bank: antigen/antibody interaction, technical aspects of blood group system			
2	Familiarity with current recommendation of method, time restriction, sample quantity and type			
3	Familiarity of current guideline for handling, accepting / rejecting specimens			
4	Familiarity with crossmatch procedure			
5	Performance of ABO and Rh typing			
6	Performance of Antibody Screening: determine positive and negative results, identification of positive screen by antibody panel, evaluation of positive antibody and subsequent procedure ie. crossmatch			
7	Direct Antiglobulin Test (Coombs): principle and procedure			
8	Indirect Antiglobulin Test (Coombs): principle and procedure			
9	Transfusion reaction workup			
10	FFP, PC, Platelet, and Neonate set-up: correct paperwork, correct labels on bags, proper expiration dates and incubator temperatures, use of scale to determine weight			
11	Knowledgeable in: maintenance of blood sterility, adherence to expiration dates, storage temperatures- maintaining logs, proper refrigerator operation and temp.			
12	Knowledge of criteria for neonatal transfusion and exchange transfusion selection of blood: age (birth to 4 mos old), selection of blood, set-up procedure label and issue			
13	Knowledge of Emergency Transfusion: selection of blood, set-up procedure, label and issue			
14	Knowledge of compatibility testing: major / minor crossmatch, identification / label of specimens, cell washer procedure (including QC/PM), sample, controls, results, incubation time/temperature, serofuge time/RPM, agglutination determination, visual aid use (light/microscope), sample retention time/place			
15	Daily reagent quality control			
16	Daily QC/PM regarding: cleaning, gloving, safety, infection control, documentation/labeling			
17	Ensures that all procedures are followed exactly for all manual procedures performed.			
18	Knowledge of procedures for resolving technical problems, blood group discrepancies, antigen testing, prewarm technique, mono-specific AHG			
19	Determination of weight of bag, minimum amount, short draw, proc., tubing clamp, sealing tubing, proper component prep. and storage			
20	Knowledge of proper procedure for Therapeutic Phlebotomy: consent, scheduling, procedure, paperwork			
21	Knowledge and complete compliance of all QC and PM, safety and infection control requirements (gloves, cleaning, labeling reagents)			
22	Knowledge of FFP, PC, and Platelet preparation, temperature requirements, operation of centrifuge, use of plasma expressor, QC and log books, time and weight requirements			
	OTHER NOT LISTED ABOVE:			

Comments:
_____
_____

Employee Signature: _____ Date: _____

Supervisor Signature: _____ Date: _____

Lab Director Signature: _____ Date: _____

INITIAL TRAINING AND COMPETENCY CHECKLIST BLOOD BANK
Instructions for Supervisor/Evaluator
- Use correct form. A sample specific for your section should be in your manual.
- Refer to competency testing policy for general information.
- Use the following symbols to indicate competence:

Y: Yes, competent
N: No, needs training
NA: Item not applicable

- If any failure to demonstrate competence is observed, the evaluator must initiate and complete a "Competency: Remediation Form". See the competency remediation procedure.
- Have employee sign and date the evaluation form indicating that he/she agrees with the evaluation

Instructions for Employee
If you feel that the training and competence evaluation is inadequate or inappropriate, ask for a conference to include the section supervisor and Lab Supervisor.

My assessment: The check boxes are all "yes" or "no". If the tech gets a "no" box checked off where it should be "yes" they are immediately referred for additional education and/or training, and then re-tested. In my experience there are few techs that fail the initial competency testing, and almost none fail the annual competency testing.

I have not seen repeat competency testing failure after reeducation and/or retraining. If this were ever to happen, you would have to call the Personnel Office and/or Human Resources Department at your hospital to ask what to do. The Personnel Office would likely have policies requiring suspension or removal of any employee that repeatedly fails competency testing.

The "yes" or "no" checkbox nature of the assessment assumes that competence is binary - all or none. In my experience competency is really a spectrum or continuum, ranging from perfect competence to perfect incompetence with infinite possibilities in between.

In my experience, competence tends to decline very slowly with age. You do not have to worry much about a tech that recently graduated from training. In order to get through training, their performance was evaluated by numerous professors. Be wary of any tech that is working past the usual social security retirement age, currently 66 years old.

Notice that in the lab where I work the form does not have checkboxes for an overall grade, not even "pass" or "fail" boxes. CLIA does not require an overall grade. All that is required is that any possible deficiencies are identified and corrected. If any deficiencies cannot be corrected, the tech cannot continue with the patient testing.

Although CLIA does not require an overall grade for the techs, your Personnel Office most likely will require you to do this. In the hospital lab where I work the Personnel Office makes us use their paperwork to give the lab techs an overall grade. Most labs assign an overall grade to the tech as part of the competency testing. If an overall grade is assigned, it may be "pass" or "fail". Alternatively, a variety of gradations may be used such as:

1. Outstanding. The tech does more work than is expected, works independently, is able to supervise other techs, and/or has skills or knowledge beyond that expected for a tech allowing the tech to do something extraordinary such as taking on work in areas a tech would not be expected to work in. The tech arrives early, leaves late and has not missed one working day in the time frame being evaluated. The tech has made no mistakes at all during the time frame being evaluated.

2. Acceptable. The tech does the amount of work expected of a tech in the time allotted, functions independently and may or may not be able to supervise other techs. The tech shows up to work on time and doesn't abuse sick leave. The tech will make a very rare mistake that doesn't affect patient care and will correct his or her own mistakes.

3. Barely acceptable. The tech may not get all the assigned work done on all days. The tech needs frequent supervision to ensure that the job is done correctly and/or all work is done. The tech may come in to work late and/or abuse sick leave on occasion, but not consistently The tech makes occasional mistakes that have to be corrected by other techs but these do not have the potential to cause patient harm.

4. Unacceptable. The tech is not able to get much work done and/or not able to function independently The tech requires constant supervision. If not constantly supervised, will not

do any work and/or will make frequent mistakes that have the potential to cause patient harm. The tech consistently comes in late and abuses sick leave. Other techs have to spend a good deal of their time correcting this tech's mistakes.

The evaluation form is filled out behind closed doors. The tech is called in to a closed door meeting with his or her supervisor and presented with the findings. The tech is asked to sign the form. There is a field on the form for the tech to write in any responses if he or she wants. The form is filed in with that tech's other competency testing documents in a folder kept in a locked file cabinet. The key to that locked file cabinet is kept secure usually by hiding the key someplace where only the Lab Supervisor and Lab Director know to find it.

Another related topic is promotion and retention of lab staff. Most of the labs I have worked at have a core membership of long term techs who have been working at that lab for many years. They tend to occupy the Lab Supervisor and section supervisor positions. This group is older, typically at least age 50, and will stay at the same lab until retirement.

As each one retires, another member of this long term group moves up to the position vacated by retirement. Hence, for this cadre, promotion occurs by the retirement of the person above them. This is not a problem when one of the section supervisors retires. The number two person in that section automatically moves up to the section supervisor position. The number three person in that section automatically moves up to the number two position, etc.

This creates a problem when the Lab Supervisor retires. The Lab Supervisor position is up for grabs and most of the section supervisors will be interested. Only one section supervisor can be promoted to the Lab Supervisor position. You must be prepared to give something of value to the section supervisors who applied for the Lab Supervisor position but were passed up.

There is a group of younger techs working in the bench level positions. They are younger and more mobile. In most labs, the retention efforts are mainly directed to the younger, more mobile lab techs.

At most of the labs I have worked at retention has been difficult. These hospitals were cash strapped and couldn't afford raises or bonuses. Other smaller perks could be offered, such as the off-site analyzer training which tends to be seen as a free vacation.

In my experience, lab tech compensation is determined by the hospital. As Lab Director you do not have much input in determining the hourly salary rates for the various positions in lab. If a valuable lab tech receives a higher paying offer from another lab, you cannot raise the hourly rate for that lab tech's position. The only way you can counteroffer is by offering to promote that lab tech to a higher paying position. In order to carry out this reshuffling, there needs to be a higher paying position vacant in lab.

If the hospital offers annual increments, it is imperative that the lab completes the paperwork in a timely manner. If this paperwork is delayed the techs will likely not receive their increments for that year. These increments will be seen as automatic by the lab techs. If you fail to give out the annual increments, this will be seen by the affected lab techs as a huge affront.

Without much to offer in the way of financial incentives for retention, the best you can do as Lab Director is to ensure a nice, happy working environment where everyone is as friendly as possible. There are numerous points to mention is this regard. In my experience it is best to allow every position in lab as much autonomy as possible. The techs can function independently, so allow them complete autonomy. If you micromanage, and take away their autonomy, it will cause resentment. If a tech makes a suggestion for improvement to the lab, take that suggestion seriously. In the majority of situations, treat the lab techs as equals, not subordinates.

Lab staff discipline and termination are among the most contentious issues in lab. No one is perfect and everyone will make an occasional mistake. The Lab Supervisor is tasked with the discipline of the lab staff and as such, it is the Lab Supervisor's judgment call if any person in lab is making significant mistakes too often.

As Lab Director I generally respect this judgment call by the Lab Supervisor. I am not a lab tech whereas the Lab Supervisor is. The Lab Supervisor knows the ins and outs of a lab tech's job and if the Lab Supervisor makes a judgment call that one of them is making too many mistakes, I will back the Lab Supervisor's decision. The only exception is if there seems to be some personal grudge involved. In that circumstance I will ask the Lab Supervisor privately if he or she is sure that the action being taken is the right thing to do.

In theory there is a long list of causes to remove an employee. Aside from mistakes this would include behavior problems, low productivity, alcohol problem, even poor morale. In reality mistakes are almost the only cause I have seen for a lab tech's removal.

Most hospital labs are short of staff and many are very short. They can't be choosey in who they employ. I have known of a lab tech who had an alcohol problem so severe that he was in and out of rehab for more than 2 years. That tech was allowed to work the entire time that he was not locked up in rehab.

I have almost never seen a lab tech removed for behavior problems. I am aware of lab techs with major mental illnesses including schizophrenia and manic depression. If the lab tech is on medication, and the mental illness is under control, they can continue to work. They cannot work if actively hallucinating or having a manic phase. Generally the tech will know the difference and call in sick if they are not able to work. The supervisor will be familiar with the tech's problems, and is usually quickly able to tell if the tech can work on days that tech comes in.

The lab tech mentioned above in the chapter on spotting a potentially suicidal employee was getting divorced, repeatedly late to work and repeatedly crying at work. The Lab Supervisor decided that this lab tech did not need mandatory referral to a Psychiatrist. This lab tech would eventually sort things out on her own, completing the divorce and moving on with her life.

In some circumstances low productivity is not a cause for removal either. I know of one older lab tech who had a stroke resulting in weakness in his right hand. He was able to return to work, but his productivity was very low, about half of what it had been before the stroke. He applied for disability retirement, but the retirement board said that he could still work and he was not disabled. He continued to work for a few more years until he reached his age based retirement. During that time, the other lab staff pitched in to help with the work, so as to make up for his low productivity.

Let's review the situation discussed in chapter 12 of the phlebotomist who switched specimens, putting the wrong patient labels on two tubes of blood. There is no question this is a huge mistake, and could easily cause patient fatalities. The hospital administrative manual states that grounds for disciplinary action include inexcusable failure to discharge duties in an efficient manner. The progressive discipline scheme is as follows:

1. Verbal warning from supervisor
2. Written warning from supervisor
3. Suspension for 2 weeks
4. Termination for cause.

The hospital administrative manual also states that if the offense is particularly serious, you can skip the first two steps and start with the third step. Although the switching of specimens is a huge mistake, let's say the phlebotomist has been a long term employee with a good track record up to this point. The Lab Supervisor decides for convenience that this can be a four step progressive discipline pathway instead of a two step progressive discipline pathway.

The progressive discipline scheme given above starts with a verbal warning. For less serious offenses, this can be a simple reminder from the Lab Supervisor of the lab's policies, for example "the lab's policies require all employees to arrive at work on time".

For a serious mistake such as switched specimens, the counseling is done in a closed-door meeting by the Lab Supervisor with the section supervisor and Lab Director present in the room. Be as nice as possible. At the minimum, you have to inform that person of the offense that person committed, the possible or actual adverse effects to patient care, the lab and/or hospital policy that has been violated, discuss how to prevent recurrences, and the consequences of further violations of that policy.

Usually, that one meeting shakes up the phlebotomist enough that they will never switch another specimen. The Lab Supervisor may want to follow up at regular intervals to see how that phlebotomist is doing. This could be done in additional closed-door meetings, and/or the Lab Supervisor can simply ask the phlebotomist in passing "Have you been remembering to check the patient wristbands while drawing?"

If that phlebotomist never again switches specimens, the problem is solved. If that phlebotomist continues to switch specimens, follow the progressive discipline procedure outlined above. Each step of the pathway involves a closed-door meeting with the person being disciplined. The meetings are conducted by the Lab Supervisor with the section supervisor and Lab Director present in the room.

Each of these meetings follows the same general outline: recite the list of offenses that person has committed, the possible or actual adverse effects to patient care, the lab and/or hospital policy that has been violated, discuss how to prevent recurrences, and the consequences of further violations of that policy.

Each step of the pathway likely has a form associated with it, e.g. written counseling form, suspension for cause form, termination for cause form. The Lab Supervisor will fill out the appropriate form, sign it and present it to the employee during or after the meeting described above. The employee may sign it or refuse to sign. Either way it is a valid document after you sign it as Lab Director. The final disposition of the form is dictated by the progressive discipline procedure. Typically the completed form ends up in the employee's competency testing folder with a copy going to the employee and another copy going to the hospital's Personnel Office.

In most hospitals the employee is allowed an appeals procedure. It is important to follow the progressive discipline procedure to the letter. If you deviate even one iota from the progressive discipline procedure, the appeals process could overturn your decisions.

No one likes to wave the axe on coworkers. It will make you extremely unpopular with the entire lab staff. If you have worked with this lab tech for many years your participation in the progressive discipline meetings will make you feel like you are Judas, the betrayer. At progressive discipline meetings I will let the Lab Supervisor do most of the talking. I will back up the Lab Supervisor as necessary, but he or she is really in charge of these meetings. As Lab Director you should make someone else wear the black hat to the extent possible.

Chapter 17 – Planning and deciding which tests to do in-house

CAP's criteria for the Clinical Laboratory Director lists strategic planning. This is defining the lab's direction and making decisions on allocating its resources to pursue this direction.

In my experience, most labs plan to stay the same forever. The next years budget is the same as last years budget with a small increment to make up for inflation. I have not seen an existing lab make a major change in direction. When labs change, it is usually in small steps. Most Lab Directors and lab management are very conservative in this regard.

Testing has changed over the years, and hospital labs have kept up with technology for the most part. When I stated in the field, neither troponin nor BNP testing was readily available to the small community hospital. They were added as they became available on the chemistry equipment in use at the typical hospital lab. Later troponin became available as a point of care test, and the hospitals I have worked at all switched troponin to point of care testing.

During the same time frame, some older tests and methodologies have been discontinued. When a test is discontinued by the manufacturer, it forces the hospital labs using that test to switch to newer methodology. In my first job out of training, I had looked at occasional blood parasite smears to rule out malaria. Now that test is obsolete and replaced by a DNA technique which is much more sensitive than the human eye. Blood parasite smears have been discontinued by most small hospital labs.

My assessment of the field is that everything is moving to waived testing. More and more tests are available as waived tests, and this seems to be the direction that everything is heading.

The decision as to which tests to send out and which tests to run in-house depends on both economic and medical considerations. If there is an overriding medical necessity for putting the test in-house you will have to do so no matter what the cost. This situation is relatively rare, and in my experience for most analytes this decision making is based on economics.

If any given analyte is sent out for testing and you are looking to bring the test in-house do the following. First, determine the medical necessity. Ask the providers that most frequently order the test what their feelings are in regard to the current arrangement. Is the turn around time fast enough? How heavily do they rely on the results of the test when evaluating patients?

If the providers want a fast turnaround time and depend heavily on the test, you are obligated to put the test in-house, otherwise you are making the decision based on economics.

Here's how to get a rough feel for the economics of testing in-house. Add up the total number of tests for that analyte sent out over the last year. Multiply this by the cost per test to figure the annual amount spent on that testing. Figure out how much the supplies and reagents would have been to do this many tests in-house. Remember to add in the costs of PT testing, controls, calibrators, tech time, etc.

I like to see the in-house testing on paper look at least 10% to 20% less expensive than send out testing before proceeding. Oftentimes there are hidden costs with in-house testing that you don't initially figure on. If the numbers come out favorable for in-house testing, then that is the way to go.

The more often a test is ordered the better the in-house testing does financially. If you put a new test in-house make sure to advertise it – send a memo to the medical staff telling them that the test is available in house with a short turn around time. Present a grand rounds on the disease associated with that particular test, etc. The more you raise awareness of the test, and/or the disease associated with that test, the more the test will be ordered, and the better that particular test will perform financially.

Chapter 18 – Other duties delegated to the Lab Director

The Lab Director is responsible for everything in lab in much the same way a captain is responsible for everything on his or her ship. I have seen literature indicating that the Lab Director has responsibility for such things as test development, the workflow in Lab, the decor on the walls, billing, keeping the internet connection up, etc. In my opinion, this is perpetuating a myth. A myth is defined as a belief that is persistent, pervasive yet unrealistic.

It is unrealistic to expect the Lab Director to do everything in Lab, such as test development, the workflow in lab, choosing the internal decor, billing, keeping the internet connection up, etc. Few hospitals do their own test development, instead the testing equipment is bought from vendors. The rest of this list is all delegated to the Lab Supervisor, billing department, hospital-wide interior decorator, Information Services Department, etc. The captain of a ship is held up to the same unrealistic expectations, and likewise delegates these duties off to multiple subordinates.

I will give lab workflow as an example. The workflow can be summarized as follows. A doctor comes in for rounds and sees a patient. The doctor tells the nurse to order a STAT serum radon level. The nurse types the order in the computer. The doctor reviews the order and verifies it in the computer using his or her electronic signature. The order is transmitted in the hospital computer to the lab. This will print out a page in the phlebotomy pick up printer. This page will include the patient name, room number, and type of tube to draw (green top).

The phlebotomist will come to the patient's bed, identify the patient, draw the patient, properly label the green top tube and return to the lab with the specimen. The tube of blood is handed off to the tech doing the testing. The test is run and the results go from the analyzer to the hospital's computer system. The results are now viewable in the patient's hospital computer chart. Since it is a STAT test the doctor is called with the results.

Essentially none of this process is under the direct supervision of the Lab Director. Some of the action involves the nurse and doctor on the ward, such that the Lab Director does not have any authority over the action. The workflow pathway is largely determined by the hospital's computer system. In other words, the hospital's computer typically has only one way to handle test requests, specimen routing, and test results such that all tests must follow this pathway. Yet the Lab Director is responsible for the entire process, from start to finish, much the same way the captain of a ship is responsible for everything on the ship.

In this circumstance, do the same thing that a ship's captain would do, optimize everything you can. Make sure that everything under your control is running smoothly and hope that the ship never sinks. If it does, you may be going down with that ship.

Several tasks are made the responsibility of the Lab Director under CLIA. This includes making sure the physical and environmental conditions of the laboratory are adequate and appropriate for the testing performed, the environment for employees is safe from physical, chemical, and biological hazards and safety and biohazard requirements are followed.

In my experience this is always delegated to the the hospital's safety office, employee health, or other similar office outside Lab. The Lab Supervisor enforces the lab's internal policies such as universal precautions. I have never seen a Lab Director taking an active role in physical or environmental issues within lab.

Essentially all clinical labs in the US are covered by the Occupational Safety and Health Administration (OSHA) regulations. These regulations require that for all toxic substances used in the workplace, the Material Safety Data Sheet (MSDS) has to be readily available in the workplace. This is usually accomplished by having each section of lab store a 3 ring binder with all the relevant MSDS sheets in the same cabinet as that section's procedure manuals.

Other OSHA regulations covering lab require that Personal Protective Equipment (PPE) be available for use and in good working order. The lab must train the staff on how to put on, use and take off the PPE. The lab must have procedures for infectious agent containment, ventilation failure, first aid, fires, emergencies and controlling the risk of exposure to chemical and biological hazards. The lab must ensure clean and sanitary conditions. Fire extinguishers, emergency eyewashes and showers must be tested on a routine basis to ensure good working order. The lab must keep a record of all workplace accidents, spills and exposures and prepare an annual summary. The lab must ensure waste disposal meets OSHA regulations. OSHA will inspect each lab annually.

OSHA does not specifically require fire drills, but recommends that they should be conducted at least annually. Most hospitals I have worked at have annual fire drills and disaster drills. These can be a fun diversion from the routine work at hand. The simplest disaster drill consists of herding all the lab staff out into a corridor deemed to be safe from tornadoes. I have been to much more elaborate drills, including mass casualty disaster drills conducted as a joint exercise between the hospital and airport. In these drills actors were painted with red paint at the airport to simulate blood then driven by ambulance to the hospital. One fire drill I went to had a "live fire" exercise whereby the trainers took the trainees into the parking lot, set fire to a barrel full of newspapers and the trainees one-by-one had to put out the fire using a fire extinguisher.

The only real mass casualty disaster I have attended to was the August 6, 1997 crash of Korean Airlines flight 801. It went down on Guam with 223 people aboard a little after 1AM. There were three Pathologists on Guam at the time of the crash. At about 3AM I was paged to come in to work at the hospital and stationed at the Blood Bank. The other two Pathologists were assigned to the site of the crash and tasked with body identification. In the first 24 hours after the crash, Blood Bank drew close to 100 blood donors. I did the donor screening and most of the donor interviews. There were 6 techs that draw the donors. We all worked non-stop at a frantic pace the first 24 hours after the crash. If anyone told me that it would be possible to do that much work in 24 hours I would not have believed them.

CLIA makes it the Lab Director's responsibility that test reports include pertinent information for test interpretation. The way I interpret this is that it means each test result must have the reference range displayed. At present, all labs are computerized such that the lab result goes from the testing equipment to the hospital's computer via some type of interface. The appearance of the lab result is thus determined by the hospital's computer and computer support personnel.

Generally, the only time the display changes is when the hospital is getting a new computer system, or lab is getting new equipment. When this happens always remind the hospital's computer support personnel that the reference range must appear next to (or at least on the same page as) the test result.

CLIA states that you must be available for consultation concerning test results and the interpretation of those results as they relate to specific patient conditions. In my experience this requirement for availability can be met by being on call (cellphone number available to the hospital operator) and does not require one to be on-site full time.

CLIA makes it the Lab Director's responsibility to ensure each employee's responsibilities and duties are specified in writing.

In my experience this is always delegated to the hospital Personnel Office, Human Resources office or other similar office. The Lab Director may have some input into writing job descriptions for the positions in lab; but once written the job descriptions are kept at the Personnel Office. For each individual employee, their job description is kept in a file folder in the Personnel Office, possibly with a copy in their competency testing file folder in Lab.

CAP's list of criteria for a clinical Lab Director lists research and development. In my 23 years in Pathology and Lab Medicine, I have only had very limited research duties. The hospital Lab Director typically sits on the hospital Institutional Review Board (IRB). Under the Code of Federal Regulations, any human subject research requires approval of the IRB of the institution where the research is to be done.

While sitting on the IRB committee, my involvement consisted of voting "yes" on all the human subjects research that the local university wanted to do at the hospital. Their projects involved counseling patients on weight loss, smoking cessation, etc. Since these projects were non-invasive, a "yes" vote as an IRB committee member was not difficult.

My only direct involvement in research was with a brain research project. My involvement ran from the late 1990s to around 2004. My participation consisted of doing autopsies on request. I had no other participation in the project. Over the course of this time, I did only about 6 autopsies for this research project. The project had a hard time getting families to consent to autopsies, and the numbers of autopsies were very low.

In my experience, most Lab Directors at community hospitals have no research duties whatsoever. Only Lab Directors at university hospitals will be expected to do research.

CAP lists educational duties in its list of criteria for a clinical Lab Director. There have not been any pathology fellows, pathology residents or medical students at any hospital I have worked at. My entire career has been at small community hospitals, not directly affiliated with an educational program. Educational duties of this nature are only expected of the Lab Director at an academic hospital. On occasion I provide some education to the Lab staff, such as reviewing pictures of urine sediment crystals, synovial crystals, blood cells, etc. at the time of PT testing or PT corrective action.

CLIA and CAP mandate that the Lab Director must select the reference laboratory. In every hospital I have worked at, the hospital lab had been affiliated with its reference lab for many years before I arrived. The only time that a hospital lab will change its reference lab is when the reference lab drops the hospital lab.

In the time I have been working on Saipan one of the reference labs, Ascent Lab of California, pulled out from the local market. This sent several labs on Saipan scrambling to find a new reference lab. Thus, in my experience the reference lab chooses to affiliate with the hospital lab, and not the other way around.

CMS requires that there is a contract in place between the hospital lab and the reference lab. Before every CMS inspection make sure you can find the contract between your lab and the reference lab. The original contract likely stipulates that it renews automatically every two years if not altered by either party. If this is the case a decades old contract is still good. However, finding a copy after that length of time is problematic. Such things tend to get lost in the sands of time.

Find a copy of this contract and set it in your office in a place where you can easily produce it if an inspector shows up unannounced. If no one at your hospital can find the contract, ask the reference lab for a copy. If the reference lab can't find the contract either, it is time to make a new contract.

CLIA and CAP mandate that the Lab Director must monitor the performance of the reference laboratory. I have seen a reference lab make a significant mistake only once in my 23 years in Pathology and Lab Medicine. This episode occurred in 2000 or 2001. At the time the technology used for Acid Fast Bacilli (AFB) culture involved incubating culture bottles. Once every day, the bottles would be tested for growth by an instrument that sticks a needle into the bottle, sucks some air out, and checks for carbon dioxide as evidence of growth.

The needle has to be cleaned very carefully, so that if one bottle has AFB in it the AFB doesn't get into the subsequent bottles that are tested with the same needle. Apparently, someone at the reference lab didn't clean this needle properly and there was a specimen positive for tuberculosis at the front end of this line of bottles to test. As a result, all subsequent bottles were contaminated with tuberculosis. One by one these bottles grew tuberculosis even though the patients whose specimens were in those bottles did not have tuberculosis (i.e. false positive tests).

A handful of false positive tuberculosis results were turned out, and several patients were told that they had tuberculosis when in fact, they really did not have tuberculosis. This problem was later identified and several corrected reports were issued, correcting AFB results from positive to negative.

When this happened I called the reference lab to express my displeasure. I also sent them a few letters and memos in regard to this episode. The reference lab was apologetic. They acknowledged that they had made a significant mistake, and promised that it would not happen again.

In my formal communication with the reference lab, they said that confidentiality issues prevented them from discussing what internal actions were being taken to prevent recurrence, or what they would do to the tech who had made the mistake.

Later, I met with officials from this lab privately. They said that they had fired the tech involved. They switched to DNA testing for AFB which does not have the same problems as the older culture technology.

In this same meeting, they asked me privately if any damage was done, and if their lab was going to get sued. I said that a handful of people got put on isoniazid and other antituberculous medications for about a month, and were then taken off of the medications when it was discovered they didn't really have tuberculosis. None of them had any complications from the treatment, and none of them was interested in suing that I knew of. Most of them were glad that they didn't really have tuberculosis.

The problem of false positive AFB results never recurred. Frankly, if it had recurred I would have very quickly been looking to switch reference labs.

Chapter 19 – How to be a Lab Supervisor

Under CLIA, the Lab Director is allowed to take on the responsibilities of several lower ranking position in lab including the clinical consultant, technical consultant, technical supervisor and general supervisor as long as you meet the personnel qualification requirements.

As mentioned before, in most labs the Lab Director and clinical consultant are the same person. Only once in my career have I also had to fill in as the Lab Supervisor. In August 2013 I was hired to "turnaround" a troubled lab in a remote area. The Lab Supervisor position had been vacant for most of the prior 2 years. When I took over the leadership role in this lab, I had to carry out both the Lab Director and Lab Supervisor work, as there was no one else available to do it.

This was a very unusual situation. In my 23 years experience in Pathology and Lab Medicine I never had to take on the Lab Supervisor position before. I am only aware of one other instance were a lab had no Lab Supervisor for an expended period of time and the Lab Director had to fill in.

As mentioned above this is allowed under CLIA. It has happened in real life and is more than just a theoretical possibility. You as Lab Director should be prepared and able to take over the Lab Supervisor position should that be necessary.

The Lab Supervisor position has been described in some detail above. The Lab Supervisor is responsible for:

1. all ordering of supplies, reagents, controls, calibrators, equipment, etc. for Lab.
2. scheduling the preventative maintenance on the lab equipment if this is not done by the section supervisors
3. scheduling for the lab techs, including scheduling of vacation time.
4. most of the budgeting including preparation of the annual budget for lab.
5. enforcing lab policies (universal precautions, arrive on time to work, etc.) on the lab staff including counseling and disciplinary actions to any tech that breaks the rules.
6. receipt of PT materials, distribution of the PT materials to the various lab sections, timely completion of the PT testing event and reporting of PT results back to the PT provider.
7. In labs without a QA coordinator, most QA work including corrective actions for PT failure falls on the Lab Supervisor.
8. assisting the Lab Director in writing Plans of Correction for inspection deficiencies.
9. competency testing of the lab staff to include remedial training and/or education.
10. day-to-day, on-site supervision of all testing personnel.

    11. assists in troubleshooting for analyzer breakdowns, and/or tests out of control.

Although I was officially the acting Lab Supervisor once in 23 years, there were several instances where the Lab Supervisor position was occupied, but the person in that position wasn't getting all of the above list done. The most critical item on the above list is the ordering of lab supplies and reagents. If the Lab Supervisor has difficulty with this, you will need to help or ask the section supervisors to help.

Several years ago, I was working at a small municipal hospital when the former Lab Supervisor left. The Blood Bank supervisor was promoted into the Lab Supervisor position. There had been little preparation for the turnover, as essentially all positions in that lab were overworked. The new Lab Supervisor didn't have much knowledge of where the Purchase Orders (PO's) and other purchasing documents are kept, how to execute a PO, etc. and also didn't have much experience with general lab inventory.

In the first few months after the Lab Supervisor position changed over, the lab ran out of several different types of reagents and supplies. Some of these were for essential tests. I would get on the phone to the Materials Management Department and beg them to procure the needed reagents and supplies as fast as possible. They would ask me for the PO number, and I'd have to go pouring through the PO manuals since the Lab Supervisor could not find the PO number.

The new Lab Supervisor was having trouble with the inventory and procurement. At this lab, inventory and procurement had always been the responsibility of the Lab Supervisor. Some of the other section supervisors might have had a better grasp on inventory and procurement, but couldn't handle budgeting or personnel issues such as scheduling. It was not possible to hire an outside Lab Supervisor. This is a small hospital lab in the middle of nowhere. Recruitment is extremely difficult, especially for the lab managerial positions.

The decision was made to unofficially split the duties of the Lab Supervisor position. The Lab Supervisor would handle all the budgeting and personnel issues, while the inventory and procurement would be split among the section supervisors. Each section supervisor would have to do the inventory and procurement work for their own section of lab. This arrangement worked out well. The section supervisors didn't mind the extra work.

If this arrangement had not worked out, there would have been two possible paths forward. The Lab Director could take over the inventory and procurement. In that hospital the added work would not have overloaded me, so this is the path I would have chosen. The other possibility is reshuffling one of the other section supervisors into the Lab Supervisor position.

If the Lab Supervisor has trouble with one item on the list of Lab Supervisor duties, follow the same approach. If the Lab Supervisor has trouble with budgeting, delegate off that part of the work to whoever in lab is good with the budgeting. If the Lab Supervisor has trouble with scheduling, delegate that off to whoever in lab is good at scheduling, etc.

If someone is new in the Lab Supervisor position, it is not uncommon for him or her to have trouble with multiple items on the list of Lab Supervisor duties. Assign the section supervisors to help him or her. Give the new Lab Supervisor a few months to try to "grow into" the position. If after a few months the Lab Supervisor is still struggling, you have to think about reshuffling someone else into that position.

Aside from the Lab Supervisor position, I have filled in for other positions as well. I spent a year working in a Veteran's Hospital that had one secretary in the Pathology Department. The days she took leave, I had to type my own reports. At first, it was disconcerting. I would go from looking at slides under the microscope to typing part of the report on the computer, back to looking at slides under the microscope, back to typing more of the report on the computer, etc.

At first, it took me almost 12 hours to examine the slides that would have only taken 8 hours with the secretary present. Within a short time I became more proficient as a typist. I could do both the slide reading and the typing within 8 hours. I would also have to answer the phones while the Secretary was on leave.

At one time or other I have filled in for virtually every other position in lab, except for phlebotomy and testing. On one instance I spent a few hours at the front desk, covering while the front desk secretary left due to a personal emergency. I occasionally have to to lift boxes up to the highest levels in the storeroom for techs that are too short or too weak to lift the heavy boxes to the top shelf.

On one occasion, a particularly rainy day, my office got muddy from various people entering with dirty shoes. I called housekeeping but they were busy mopping up all the other mud in the hospital. After the working day was over, I ended up mopping my own office.

Chapter 20 – Pathologist hiring, orientation, competency testing and retirement

In my experience Pathologist hiring is even more difficult than lab tech hiring. For most of my 23 year career in Pathology and Lab Medicine I have been solo. The hospital where I was working at the time had hired Pathologists twice, once in 2000 and again in 2008. There were no other Pathologists in that municipality so hiring by word of mouth was not an option. Advertisements were placed in the Pathology journals – CAP Today, AJCP and Laboratory Medicine. In 2008 advertisements were also placed online.

In both instances there was only one applicant. In each instance the applicant was vetted by the usual state licensure process and hospital privileging process. The applicant's credentials were verified, and the applicant was licensed and privileged.

The Pathologist hired in 2000 was Dr. B. He started work in August, 2000. Immediately after staring work Dr. B began arguing with everyone in the lab. He argued with the Lab Supervisor as to whether the Lab Supervisor or the Pathologist has more authority in lab. These arguments occurred on a daily basis in public areas within the lab. He argued loudly and daily with the histotechs about the quality of the slides. After 2 months of this, Dr. B. resigned and went back where he came from.

The Pathologist hired in 2008 was Dr. W. Immediately after starting work, Dr. W. began having problems of such a nature that the hospital Medical Director mandated that Dr. W. should see the hospital Psychiatrist. The hospital Psychiatrist said that Dr. W. could not work and needed to take sick leave. The problem is that Dr. W. just stared work, and does not have any sick leave saved up. Dr. W. left on unpaid leave time, and never returned.

When it comes to Pathologist hiring, I am batting zero. This is why I was solo for so many years. You may want to take my Pathologist hiring recommendations above with a grain of salt due to my dismal track record. I like to think that the problem is a nationwide shortage of Pathologists. There is anecdotal supporting information for a Pathologist shortage, such as large numbers of vacant

Pathologist positions in desirable locations.

In terms of orientation, a Pathologist should only need orientation to the particulars of the new lab where he or she will be working. The computer system tends to be the most troublesome feature for a new Pathologist. If you are using a computer system the new Pathologist is not used to, it may take a great deal of orientation. Other particulars such as work flow may vary slightly from one lab to the next. The menu of immunostains available also varies from lab to lab and may take some getting used to. However, tissue diagnosis is the same everywhere, and should not require orientation.

As Lab Director you will supervise anatomic pathology and cytopathology. This is a little different than directing the clinical lab in that you are supervising other physicians. It also differs in that the interpretations of a slide are very subjective, whereas the results turned out by an analyzer are cut and dry – the test is either positive or negative, or else it generates a number, with no subjective interpretation. Thus, evaluating the performance of a Pathologist and/or Cytopathologist is harder than evaluating the performance of a lab tech.

The best advice I can give is as follows. All anatomic pathology and cytopathology diagnoses are interpretive opinions. No one person can claim that their opinion is the gold standard. In my experience, there is a huge amount of variation in slide interpretation among different pathologists. You must be very tolerant of every other pathologist's interpretation.

Some labs mandate a 10% lookback on the slides signed out by each Pathologists in the group. There is a small allowable rate of error. In most of these labs a "major error" rate of 1% is allowed. However, even the definition of a major error is subjective.

I have seen biopsy cases so difficult that a group of nine pathologists split three ways – 4 wanted a malignant diagnosis, 4 wanted a benign diagnosis and one was noncommittal. The case was sent out in consultation. The consultants equivocated and recommended re-biopsy. Which if any of this group made a major error in interpretation?

In my experience most practices do not do retrospective review of the pathology and cytology slides. In these labs, the evaluation of the pathologists is done based on complaints received and rates of revised (corrected) diagnoses. Even this is problematic, as one patient can file multiple unjustified complaints on a Pathologist. Pathology cases tend to be amended after the fact to add results of outside tests. If the computer adds these cases to the list of revised cases, it will make the rate of revision look much worse than it otherwise would be.

The bottom line is that when dealing with subjective interpretations, there is no gold standard. All performance measurements are relative.

Most people think of competence being all-or-none, like a light switch which can only be in the off or the on position. In reality there is a continuum or spectrum ranging from perfect competence to perfect incompetence with infinite possibilities in between. In my experience there are a few warning signs:

1. The practitioner is practicing beyond the usual age of retirement for the specialty. For Pathology the usual retirement age is 66 or 67.
2. The practitioner has medical problems, especially medical problems that would compromise cognition or vision
3. The practitioner would like to retire, but is compelled to continue working for financial

reasons
4. The practitioner is out of touch with the latest developments in the specialty, uses outdated terminology, and only has the minimum Continuing Medical Education (CME) to meet licensure requirements.
5. Multiple instances in a short time of the practitioner making a diagnosis on a slide that is completely different from all other Pathologists looking at the same slide.
6. The practitioner progressively slows down, getting less and less work done in an 8 hour day. As a result more and more work is delegated to the younger Pathologists. This work slowdown runs its course over many years, such that few people will notice until it is in a very advanced state. You will look back over the past several years, and wonder how this practitioner got away with doing so little work for so many years.

Of the above warning signs, number 5 is the most important. It indicates loss of skills and abilities. The CMS defines competency as the ability of personnel to apply their skill, knowledge, and experience to perform their duties correctly. Implied but not stated is that loss of these abilities indicates incompetence. I have also seen incompetence defined as "too many mistakes too fast".

The Joint Commission (TJC) requires Ongoing Professional Practice Evaluation (OPPE) for all physicians. If you are Lab Director of a hospital lab you will have to fill out an OPPE form for each Pathologist at least every 6 months. Annual review is not frequent enough to be "ongoing". If you are Lab Director of an outpatient lab that is not TJC certified, you are not required to fill out OPPE forms.

A Focused Professional Practice Evaluation (FPPE) is similar but only occurs when there is a triggering event. Triggers include a Pathologist arrives new to your hospital, an existing Pathologist applies for increased privileges, and/or a Pathologist has made one or more mistakes significant enough to trigger an FPPE. An FPPE is a one-time event which does not recur. Otherwise an FPPE is similar to a OPPE.

The OPPE form typically has fill in the blank boxes and/or checkboxes for workload, timeliness and competency. After completing the OPPE form you will need to check a box for overall grading as "pass" or "fail". See the form on the next page.

MY LAB				MY PROCEDURE MANUAL			
Ongoing Practitioner Performance Evaluation (OPPE) Form							
Provider:			ID #:			Department: Pathology	
Status:			Department Chairman:				
Specialty: Pathology							
		Most Current 6-mo. Period					
Indicator	1H 2014	2H 2014	1H 2015	2H 2015	6-month Thresholds		
					Exceeds	Meets	Below
Number of Cases - Pathology							
Number of Cases - Cytology							
Number of Cases - Autopsies							
Percent major disagreement at retrospective review					0%	< 1%	1% or more
Correlation of Outside Consultation with Pathologist's Diagnosis					> 95%	95%	< 95%
Surgical Pathology Report completed w/in 2 days					> 97%	97%	< 97%
Cytology Report completed w/in 3 days of receipt of specimen					> 97%	97%	< 97%
Validated Patient Complaints					0	1-3	> 3
Validated Staff Complaints					0	1-3	> 3

Overall Grade	Pass	Fail	Signature of practitioner	Signature of Department Chair
1H 2014				
2H 2014				
1H 2015				
2H 2015				

I have seen cases where the workload is zero for a particular specimen type. In general, no action can be taken against the practitioner for low or nonexistent workload. If the turn around time is prolonged, the usual result is a brief motivational talk with the Pathologist involved.

The TJC mandates that you evaluate competency, but has no specific requirement on how to measure it. In some institutions it is measured by retrospective review of cases. However this is not mandatory, and other performance measures can be chosen such as complaints received and rates of revised (corrected) diagnoses.

If your lab is doing retrospective review of cases and finds one or more Pathologist with the percent of cases having reviewer disagreement exceeding the allowable threshold, this will trigger close scrutiny. Look at the slides for the cases that have fallen out to referee them. After reviewing these cases, refer any discrepant cases back to the original signing Pathologist. Ask the original signing Pathologist to reconsider his or her diagnosis and consider issuing an amended pathology report.

If the original signing Pathologist does not reconsider, but you and the reviewing Pathologist feel strongly about the case, you will need to have the case reviewed further. If you are in a large group, show the slides to the entire group and vote on the diagnosis. A simple majority vote wins. If you are in a small group, send the case out to a subspecialist for refereeing.

A few minor disagreements are common; nothing further needs to be done. If one or more major disagreement is identified, you will need to call that Pathologist into your office and have a long talk. Ask how this happened and how it can be prevented in the future. Suggest to that Pathologist that you are always open for consultations, and can review any case(s) that Pathologist wants reviewed.

If this is an isolated instance, nothing further needs to be done. If it recurs, there are a number of options to consider. You may need to assign that Pathologist a proctor to review some or all of that Pathologist's cases before sign-out. You are in effect demoting an Attending level physician to a Fellowship level, but this may be necessary given the circumstances. If the Pathologist is having medical problems, request that Pathologist to submit medical clearance from his or her physician. If that Pathologist is still in the probationary period, extend the probationary period if possible.

If the problem is resolved by any of the above means, no further action needs to be taken. If the excessive rate of major discrepancies continues, you are going to have to call that Pathologist in for a long series of talks about retirement. Give a retirement pep talk: You are really going to love retirement, it is so much fun to be retired. I retired from Pathology to Lab Director work and love it. You can spend more time with your grandchildren.

The needs of the patient take priority over the needs of this Pathologist. If you can't talk this Pathologist into retirement and the Pathologist still has an excessive rate of major discrepancies, the next step is to take the matter to the hospital Medical Director. The Medical Director will likely not have much understanding of pathology and the situation may require quite a bit of explaining. You may have to meet more than once with the Medical Director to adequately explain the situation. Provide copies of all the documents related to the retrospective reviews, major discrepancies, etc. to the Medical Director.

Any seasoned Medical Director will have had prior experience dealing with physician performance issues, and will have a good idea of what to do. The Medical Director will call in that Pathologist for a very unpleasant series of meetings. You as Lab Director will likely have to sit in on the majority of these meetings.

The hospital Medical Director can force a retirement, typically on threat of summary suspension of clinical privileges. The Medical Director will not be bluffing. I have seen at least one case in which the hospital Medial Director actually did follow through on the threat of summary suspension for a Pathologist that refused retirement. This is a horrible way for an elderly Pathologist to end his or her career but in some cases it can't be avoided.

Doing this to a colleague can be heartbreaking, especially if you have worked with that Pathologist for many years. It will make you feel like Judas, the betrayer, but it is necessary given the circumstances.

I will give the example of Dr. S. an elderly Pathologist I was working with at my first job after graduating training in 1996. Dr. S. was born around 1923. He had three wives, two divorces, and a total of 8 children (3 children with his first wife, 3 children with his second wife, and 2 children with his third wife). He had lost all his savings to divorce, alimony and child support.

He had no savings for retirement and for financial reasons continued working as a Pathologist into his late 70s. Sometime in 1999 he had an episode of acute angle glaucoma in his right eye. He went out on sick leave for a few weeks. There was some debate as to whether he should be allowed to return to work. He had some loss of vision in the right eye, correctable to about 20/60. The ophthalmologist did not know the visual acuity necessary to be a Pathologist. The literature does not state any minimum visual acuity for working as a Pathologist.

While Dr. S. was out on leave his situation was discussed a number of times between the Pathologists and Lab Director. I was in a Pathologist position, and had no strong feelings either way as to whether he should or should not be allowed to return. The Lab Director for that hospital had worked with Dr. S. for many years and was a close friend. The decision was made to allow Dr. S. to return to work.

Dr. S. wanted to keep working, and was allowed to keep working. In the subsequent 6 months he made significant mis-steps. One involved a mastectomy for carcinoma. He correctly called the breast lesion as an infiltrating ductal carcinoma. He called one lymph node positive for metastatic carcinoma. The patient was referred to a different hospital for chemotherapy. As is the usual practice, the pathologists at the referral hospital reviewed the case. They called the lymph node negative for carcinoma.

This same lymph node slide has been looked at by over a dozen Pathologists and all Pathologists except for Dr. S. have called that lymph node negative for metastatic carcinoma. The block was recut and stained with immunos, and over a dozen pathologists called the immuno slides negative for metastatic carcinoma.

Dr. S. had two other mis-steps in the first 6 months after his episode of acute angle glaucoma. In one of these he mistook an endocervical adenocarcinoma in-situ for adenoma malignum. In the other, he mistook a reactive lymph node for lymphoma.

Dr. S. was forced to retire from his Pathologist position. He was around 78 years old at the time. He subsequently got a desk job as a Lab Director in a different state. He worked as a Lab Director for another 8 years until he got Parkinson's disease and became wheelchair-bound. He was around 86 years old when this happened. He wanted to continue working, but was forced to retire from that Lab Director position because he could no longer carry out the duties of the job position.

The point of this story is that there are people in this world who will continue to work until well after it is obvious that they can no longer do the job. Such a person has no insight into their own condition and will continue working until forced to stop. Your mission is to help them to retire. They may not like it, but at this point retirement is in their best interest and in your best interest as well.

The above story is an extreme example of a retirement done the wrong way by the retiree. Most Pathologist retirements I have seen have been done more or less the right way. The right way to retire, as I see it, is a gradual cutting back on work to match the slow declines in cognitive function and vision due to aging.

When I started my first job after graduating training in 1996 the Lab Director at that hospital was in his mid 60s. He was the sharpest Pathologist I had ever seen. Over the course of the next few years, he would lose some of his brilliance but was still very sharp. He retired from tissue exams in the year 2000 while in his late 60s. At that time he retained several Lab Directorships, including one at a major hospital lab.

He continued losing sharpness over the ensuing years. He retired from the hospital Lab Director position in 2005 while in his mid 70s. He retained Lab Directorships at a few small clinics. These were very easy desk jobs that consisted of coming in a few times a month to sign papers for a few hours.

At present, he is an extremely elderly, frail gentleman in his early 80s, almost completely lacking the sharpness and energy he had 18 years prior. He has cut back to one small clinic Lab Directorship. He would like to retire from that position, but the clinic can't find a replacement.

This story, of a slow cutting back of one's work, is typical of a Pathologist's retirement. Less common is the situation where one stops work completely when one becomes eligible for Social Security retirement, currently the 66th birthday. I have known a few Pathologists who took this approach, ending their career abruptly, like a door slammed shut on their 66th birthday.

Chapter 21 – How to go through the inspection process

    A. How to pick an inspecting agency and prepare for the inspection

In the US all medical labs fall under CLIA. For labs doing moderate and/or high complexity testing, inspections are carried out by CMS, or any inspecting agency with deemed status. CMS will call its visit to your lab a "survey" but everyone else calls it an "inspection".

The deemed status inspecting agencies include CAP, COLA and TJC. The States of New York and Washington also have deemed status. These accrediting organizations have been "deemed" by CMS as having standards and inspections that meet or exceed the Medicare/Medicaid Conditions of Participation (CoP). Labs inspected by the "deemed status" inspecting agencies are not subject to the CMS inspection and certification process since they are assumed to already meet minimum Medicare and Medicaid requirements. After successful completion of the inspection a CMS Certificate of Compliance, CAP Certificate of Accreditation, or similar documentation is issued.

The difficulty level in passing an inspection from any of the inspecting agencies is roughly the same. The deemed status inspecting agencies must meet CLIA requirements at a minimum but can also add their own requirements. Hence CMS is probably the easiest, most minimal inspection to pass. For small labs with little staffing, CMS inspections are likely to be the best choice. For larger labs with more staffing, consider CAP inspections which are seen as more prestigious.

Some insurers will only reimburse to labs accredited by CAP. Before you pick your inspector, make sure you discuss with your billing department as to what the local insurance companies require for reimbursement.

The FDA and AABB only inspect Blood Bank, not the entire lab. The AABB does not have "deemed status" with the FDA such that if you sign up for AABB inspections you will still get FDA inspections. Elect for FDA inspections alone if you are heading up a small lab with limited resources. If you are in a large Blood Bank with a great deal of staff, consider adding AABB inspections for the prestige. The process of preparation, inspection and remediation of deficiencies is the same for FDA and AABB inspections as for the general lab inspections described below.

To prepare for the inspection, go through your lab the way the inspector would. Look at all the procedure manuals. Are the manuals complete? Is there a procedure for every test done in-house? Are all procedures signed by the Lab Director? For CAP inspections, were the manuals signed within the last 2 years?

Look at your lab's proficiency testing. The inspectors will generally only look back at the last 2 years of data. How many failures did you have in the last 2 years? Do all PT failures have an acceptable corrective action?

Go through the lab general documents and each of the sections – chemistry, hematology, Blood Bank, urinalysis, etc. Look through the procedure manuals, QA logs, etc. as if you were an inspector. This does not have to be as formal as a "mock inspection" or self-inspection, but should at least cover the basics.

This will give you some idea if you are ready or not for the inspection. If you are ready, then it is just a matter of keeping things in order in the time left before the inspection. If there is still much work to be done, you will be staying late, or very late at work trying to get it all caught up before the inspection.

In my experience the two most common citations involve expired reagents and storage of excessive amounts of paper records in lab. While preparing for the inspection, assign each section supervisor to inventory their section for expired reagents. These expired reagents must be replaced with in-date reagents by the time of the inspection. If there are numerous boxes of paper records being stored in lab, check which records are old enough to be shredded. Shred any boxes of documents that are beyond the required retention time. If you have many boxes of documents that are too recent to shred, you can send them to off-site storage as long as they are easily retrievable from that storage and safe from destruction. Make sure any boxes of records present in lab are off the floor and not blocking fire exits.

First impressions are important. If the CMS inspectors come into your lab and find it dirty, with boxes of records stacked up to the ceiling, they will not think too highly of your lab. This could result in a citation in and of itself. Try to keep the number of boxes of records to a minimum. Try to have the lab cleaned to the extent possible. Usually the hospital Housekeeping Department is called in during the run-up to the inspection to give lab a thorough cleaning. In most labs I have worked at, the lab gets its floors waxed once every 2 years in the run-up to the inspection. If the floors have not been waxed in years, this will go a long way toward making the lab look cleaner.

Here is a tip that a CMS inspector once gave me. The inspector is only allowed to ask for the last 2 years of lab documentation, which should correspond to the documentation since the last inspection. However, if you leave lab QC manuals sitting out that are more than 2 years old, the inspector is allowed to look at them. If you had a QC failure 3 years ago, and the inspector missed it on the last inspection, the only way it could be caught is if you leave the manual in plain sight at the next inspection. Thus when preparing for the inspection, try to only leave the last 2 years of documentation in plain sight. Keep the older documentation locked in a cabinet where it can't be seen, but can be retrieved if necessary.

B. The day of the inspection

The day the inspectors come, they will usually take over your breakroom as their office area. Make sure to have a large breakfast and lunch served. At the minimum, you do not want them to be hungry during the inspection. They will come and look through all your documentation. They may or may not watch one or more tech do the testing. They may or may not follow specimens as they are processed through you lab. They may take a quick tour of other parts of the hospital – morgue, fingerstick glucose testing in other wards, the computer center, etc.

At the end of the inspection you and the hospital administrator will be called for the summation meeting. This meeting is sometimes referred to as an "exit interview". In this meeting the inspectors will recite their list of findings. Many of these will be recommendations. A recommendation is a suggestion as to how to improve your lab. You are not obligated to follow the recommendations; you can continue doing things the same way if you want.

In regard to the recommendations, inspections are very useful. Outside lab experts are coming to your lab and looking at how your lab does things. Their input is valuable. The CMS inspectors are likely to be as current as possible on the latest developments in the lab field, and their recommendations should be taken seriously.

A citation is a finding that you are obligated to correct in order to continue being certified by the inspecting agency. Almost all labs will get a few small citations on any given inspection. From what I have heard, the inspectors feel obligated to give at least one citation so as to justify their inspection. In a CMS inspection the citations are divided into three levels of deficiency. I will discuss these at length later in this chapter. In increasing order of severity they are:

1. standard level deficiency
2. condition level deficiency
3. immediate jeopardy

Pay close attention to everything the inspectors say in the exit interview. You will need to respond to the citations. Make sure you are very clear on the citations. If you don't understand a citation, ask for further clarification. For any complex citation, I would ask the inspectors for suggestions on how to correct the citation.

In the exit interview, the inspectors will rattle off a list of findings. It is important to maintain your composure in this meeting and be as nice as possible. The inspectors may give off a long list of things you have done wrong, but it is not a personal attack. They are just doing their jobs. Avoid arguments with the CMS inspectors. If you disagree with the inspectors on a finding, it may be best to approach them after the meeting is over to discuss that particular finding further. I am aware of one physician Nursing Home Director who was fired for getting into an argument with CMS inspectors at the exit interview.

After the end of the inspection you will receive a copy of the inspection paperwork with the list of citations. Your lab will need to prepare a response to each citation, usually within 10 days of receiving them. You may or may not receive an accompanying letter with the following verbatim from CMS on how to make a plan of correction.

> The acceptable evidence of correction that you must provide to CMS must include at a minimum:
>
> 1. documentation showing what corrective action(s) have been taken for patients found to have been affected by the deficient practice;
> 2. an explanation of how the laboratory has identified other patients having the potential to be affected by the same deficient practice and what corrective actions(s) has been taken;
> 3. a description of the measures that have been put into place or systemic changes made to ensure that the deficient practice does not recur;
> 4. a description of how the corrective actions are being monitored to ensure the deficient practice does not recur.

Although this is the verbatim from CMS, there is much more to making a Plan of Correction than the skeletal outline given above. If you followed the instructions from CMS given above, and did no further work, the CMS inspectors would almost certainly reject your Plan of Correction when you send it in to CMS. I will go in great detail below about how to make a passable Plan of Correction.

In theory, the Lab Supervisor is responsible for all corrective actions in Lab, including responses to inspection citations. In reality, the Lab Supervisor and Lab Director write the responses together.

C. How to fill out CMS form 2567 and write a Plan of Correction

Here is an example of the form you will receive if inspected by the CMS and found to have citations. This is form CMS-2567 Statement of Deficiencies and Plan of Correction:

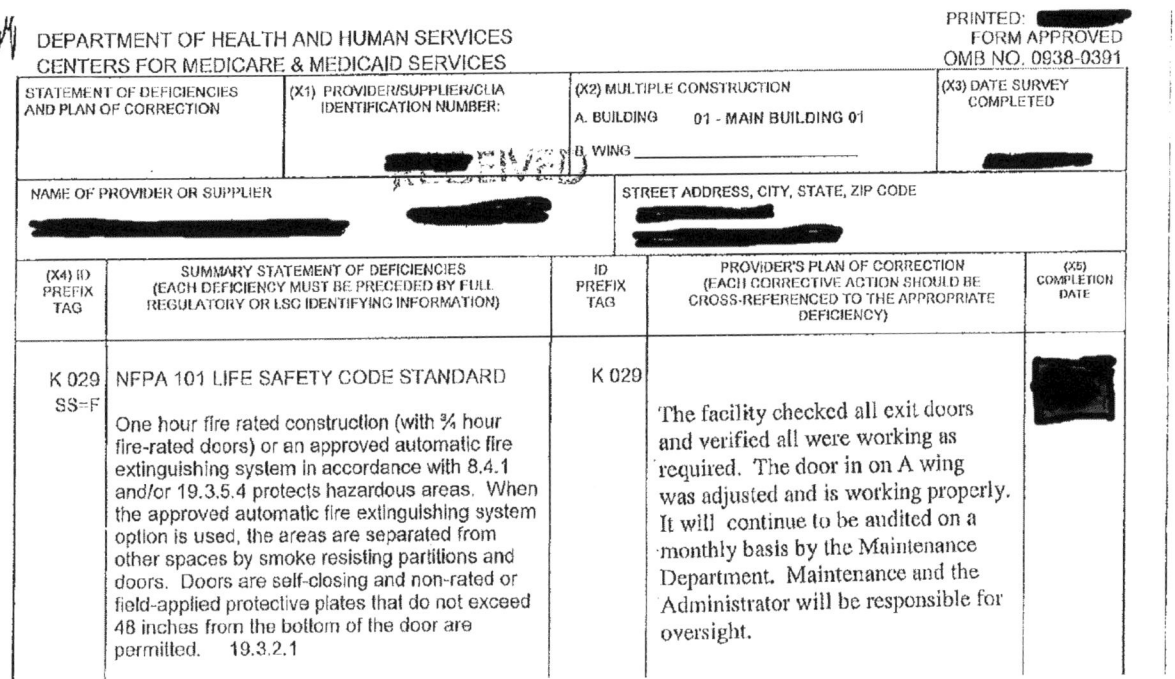

In the above example, the facility has been cited for violating the fire code because one fire door is not working properly. The left column under the header "Summary Statement of Deficiencies" should contain a description of the problem written in plain language. The inspector should have explained the citation to you at the exit interview. If you are not clear on the citation, you should be able to call the inspector at the inspector's office and ask for more explanation of the deficiency.

As with all corrective actions, the plan of correction must state how the lab has fixed the problem or plans to fix the problem, This could involve buying new equipment, new supplies, or could involve changing the lab's procedures or processes (i.e. a "systemic change" meaning the lab is changing the way it does things). There must be a time frame for completing the corrective action, preferably within 60 days but not to exceed 12 months from the last day of the inspection.

The corrective action must include a plan to monitor the situation to ensure there are no future recurrences of the problem. This often entails adding the cited problem area to the monthly quality assurance reviews. If the problem has the potential to affect patient lab results, there must be a statement that patients were not adversely affected, or documentation as to how the lab is attempting to identify and correct any possible adverse patient effects.

In the CMS literature there is no requirement for naming the person who is responsible for making the corrections and ensuring that there are no recurrences of the problem. If you are going to name the responsible party in the Plan of Correction, it is best to designate that person by title (e.g. Lab Director) and not by name (e.g. Dr. Dauterman). If the position changes over (e.g. I retire) all of the form 2567 responses that name me would have to be changed to reflect the name of the new Lab Director.

In the example above, the citation is relatively minor and easy to fix. The facility fixed the fire door in question and verified that all fire doors were working. The facility will continue to monitor the fire doors on a monthly basis to make sure that they keep working. The response was typed into the right column under the header "Provider's Plan of Correction". The estimated date of completion of the corrective action is put in the far right column under the header "Completion Date". If there are multiple citations, repeat the same process for each citation.

If your lab received a large number of citations, writing the responses can seem like a daunting task. If you look at the big picture, you may get overwhelmed. Try to look at it one citation at a time. Each plan of correction may be a single small step, but if you put all the steps together you will get through the process of writing the plans of correction. If you have difficulty writing a response to one or more citation, you are allowed to call in consultants, call for advice from the supervisors of surrounding labs, etc. You will become more proficient at writing corrective actions the more you do it. After you have been through several inspections, writing the corrective actions will seem routine and unexciting.

The fire door citation in the example above typifies a very minor citation for a lab. It is an example of a "standard level deficiency". This is the lowest of the three levels of deficiency. This level of deficiency occurs when the lab violates a standard but there is no risk of patient harm and the deficiency does not limit the lab's ability to furnish safe and effective services. In the example above, the fire door citation does not relate to the lab testing per se. The inspectors pay particular attention to details related to the health and safety of the employees, such that this type of citation is very common.

Here is another example of form CMS-2567 Statement of Deficiencies and Plan of Correction:

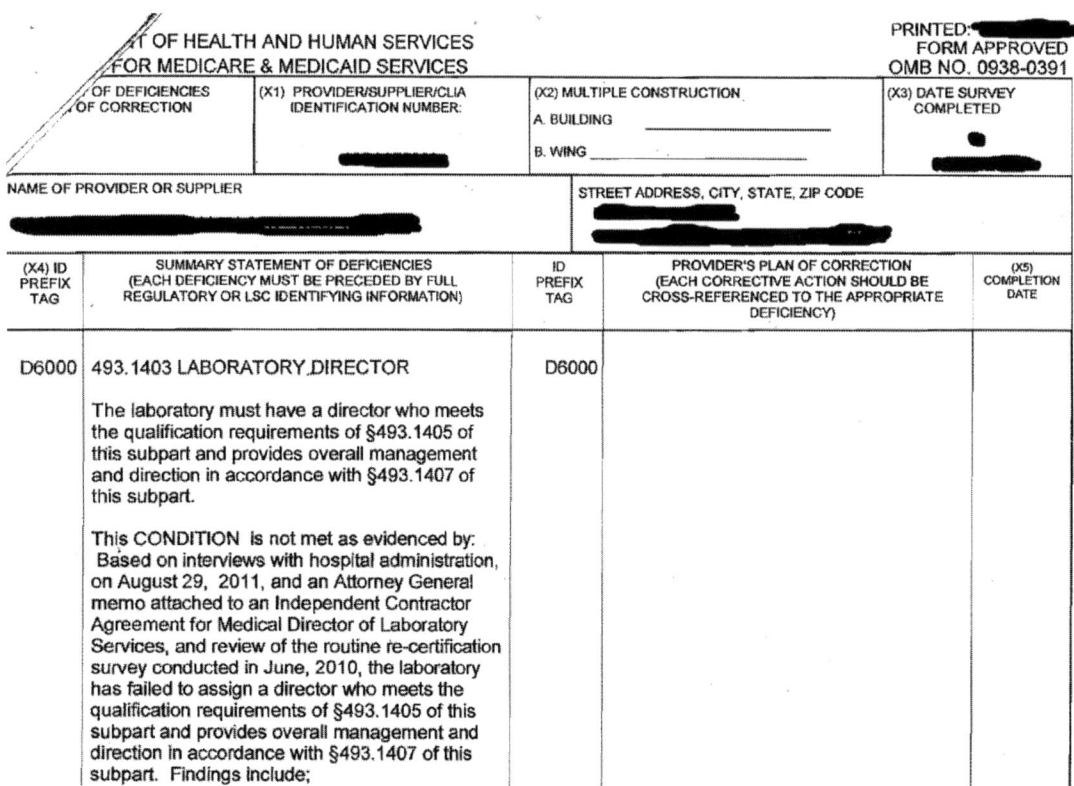

This citation is for a lab that left the Lab Director position vacant for more than one year. Per CLIA, the Lab Director position can only be left vacant for 30 days. From talking with the CMS inspectors, they consider this to be the single worst offense a lab can commit.

In the case of this lab, CMS gave the lab a type of citation called a "condition level deficiency". This is the middle of the three levels of deficiency. It means that the lab was not meeting the conditions for participating in Medicare. Condition level deficiencies limit the lab's ability to furnish safe and effective services but do not represent an immediate threat to the patients.

In the case of the vacant Lab Director citation given above, the CMS additionally gave an Immediate Jeopardy citation to this lab's hospital. This is the highest of the three levels of deficiency. An Immediate Jeopardy citation means that the CMS feels the situation is a serious and immediate risk to the life and/or safety of the patients at that hospital.

The process of corrective action is the same. The lab made a plan to hire a Lab Director and followed through on hiring a Lab Director. They hired me. This is the lab that I was hired to "turnaround" in August, 2013. My presence at that lab mitigated the greatest deficiency, and I worked very hard to correct the other problems in that lab. In the subsequent CMS inspection in December, 2013 this lab had only two minor citations.

The point is not that I fly in like Superman to fix up labs. The point is that all corrective actions follow the same process, from the most minor citation (one stuck fire door) to the worst possible citation for a lab (no Lab Director for more than a year).

In both examples of form 2567 given above, the stuck fire door and the vacant Lab Director position, there was no potential for patient harm. In other words, these deficiencies did not adversely affect patient care. If there was a potential for patient harm the Plan of Correction would need additional work. You would need to issue corrected reports for any erroneous test results and determine if the change in test results would have made a difference in patient care. You are required to inform CMS of the findings, even if you don't like what you find.

I will give an example of how this works using the nonexistent test serum radon levels and its mythical association with lung cancer. Let's say your lab was found at a CMS inspection to be out of control for serum radon levels and turning out levels too low. You have done 1000 tests in the time serum radon levels were out of control. You get the test into control, retest these 1000 specimens and find they were all too low. You have to issue a corrected report for each of these 1000 specimens. Even worse, 100 were originally false negatives. They were reported as negative, but on retest are above the action level (i.e. positive).

CLIA requires that you promptly notify the person ordering the test and, if applicable, the individual using the test results of reporting errors. The reference for this is 42 CFR §493.1291. This is interpreted as requiring a phone call to the provider to inform him or her of the change in test results.

Your lab will be making 1000 phone calls to inform the providers of the corrected test results. The providers in question will be unhappy to find that they have received erroneous test results. For 100 of those patients, you will be correcting the report from negative to positive. The providers will be even more upset in this circumstance, as it will change the clinical approach to the patient.

You are required to identify any patient that could potentially have been harmed, document that there was no harm to those patients or try to mitigate the harm to the extent possible. The way that most people interpret this is that you only have to follow up on the 100 patients that had false negative tests.

You do not need to follow up the other 900 that had a slight change in test result, but are still negative. This means that you are going to be pulling 100 charts from medical records and reviewing them all to make sure that none of the patients got lung cancer.

The effort described so far (1000 retests, 1000 phone calls, 100 chart reviews) is a huge amount of work. It would have been much easier to keep the serum radon levels in control in the first place. Hence, this is why it is so important to make sure your techs never turn out test results unless controls are in for that run or day. The cleanup afterward can involve a huge amount of work, and is a huge headache.

It gets worse from there. Let's say you pull the 100 charts from medical records and find that 3 of these patients developed lung cancer within two years of the false negative serum radon levels. Two of these three patients have passed away from lung cancer. The patient population is older, and lung cancer is so common in the elderly that if you pick 100 older people and follow them for two years it is not unlikely that 3 of them will get lung cancer.

The problem is that in this case, the 3 that got lung cancer had a false negative serum radon level from your lab in the two years before the lung cancer diagnosis. If you had turned out a positive serum radon level, these 3 patients might have gotten worked up for lung cancer, and it might have been caught earlier. The CMS inspectors are likely to interpret this as serious patient harm or patient fatalities from the testing in your lab. You have just taken a huge step toward regulatory closure of your lab.

The temptation is to try to cover up the bad outcomes. If your lab is under regulatory scrutiny, the CMS inspectors will be watching you very carefully. They will likely come unannounced, interview your staff privately, and go through your medical records department as they see fit. You will likely get caught if you try to conceal information from the CMS inspectors. If you get caught concealing information, that is another big step towards regulatory closure of your lab and now the CMS inspectors will start thinking about banning you. Thus it is in your best interest to self-report any untoward information you uncover. Let the chips fall where they may and take your lumps.

After you complete all the responses, mail the form back to the inspecting agency. Include all relevant documentation, such as copies of revised procedures, invoices for newly purchased equipment, etc. This can be mailed, FAXed or scanned and E-mailed back to the inspecting agency. The form 2567 is due back 10 days after you receive it.

If the citations are few and small, the inspecting agency will likely accept the responses, and you will then receive your notice of renewal. If your lab is having multiple small problems, your responses will be scrutinized more carefully. One or more of the initial responses may be rejected in which case you have to modify the rejected responses and send them in again.

If your facility is having significant problems, you may be asked to file a formal Plan of Correction (PoC). When making a PoC you have to respond to all the deficiencies in form 2567. In addition, you will be expected to examine your lab's methods, processes, and/or systems to identify what is not working or not consistent with current regulations. In other words, you are expected to re-think the whole way your lab does business and conducts its operations. Needless to say CMS only mandates this on a lab if it thinks there is something seriously wrong with that lab.

You will need to send your PoC in to CMS in addition to the form 2567. The PoC is due 24 days after you are requested to prepare it. Both the PoC and the form 2567 are subject to multiple rounds of revision, so as to meet CMS approval.

In some situations a lab may be asked to file a Credible Allegation of Compliance (CAoC) with CMS. The CAoC is very similar to a PoC with a few minor differences. The CAoC is typically used for more serious citations (condition level deficiencies or Immediate Jeopardy deficiencies) while the PoC is more often used for minor citations (standard level deficiencies). The corrections must be completed by the day of signing of a CAoC whereas with a PoC it is acceptable to list future dates for completion of the corrections. If there are no Immediate Jeopardy citations, the CAoC is due 45 days from the last day of inspection. If the lab has one or more Immediate Jeopardy citations, the CAoC is due 23 days from the last day of inspection. Otherwise a CAoC and a PoC are similar.

Here is an example of a form you can use if you ever get requested to make a Plan of Correction:

	Plan of Correction Form		
Provider Name:		Phone:	
Provider Contact for follow-up:		Fax:	
Contact phone:		Email:	
Address:	Provider NPI#		Date:

Finding (State the Problem)	Corrective Action Steps (How will this problem be corrected?)	What systems changes will be made to ensure this situation and others like it do not occur again?	Responsible Party	Time Line
				Implementation Date:
				Implementation Date:
				Implementation Date:
				Implementation Date:

Accepted _____ Not Accepted _____ Date _____ Initials _____ Revision Due _____

The next higher level of CMS oversight on a lab involves a directed Plan of Correction. The difference between the PoC described above and a directed PoC is that CMS mandates a directed PoC on you. You do not have much input in a directed PoC. This generally happens to a lab that proves incapable of making its own PoC.

Avoid the temptation to put little effort into making your own PoC simply because CMS will do it for you. You are much better off making your own PoC since you will have more control over the process. If CMS has to make a directed PoC for you, it is likely to be much more onerous.

The next higher level of CMS oversight involves a series of re-inspections on a lab. These re-inspections are typically done to ensure enforcement of a PoC or CAoC; hence a PoC or CAoC is typically in place before the re-inspections begin. The lab without a Lab Director referred to above had at least 3 re-inspections between its August, 2012 regular inspection and the next regular inspection 2 years later. In this situation, the CMS is sending personnel on-site to the lab similar to what the lab is lacking. However, this is not a regulatory takeover of the lab in the conventional sense. The CMS can't station Lab Directors permanently at a lab, and the CMS will expect a lab to correct its problems on its own.

If all the above fails to correct the problems in a lab, CMS has the authority to close down a lab. This is done by revocation of the CMS Certificate of Compliance. In theory a lab could continue to operate if its Certificate of Compliance is revoked. The lab wouldn't be able to bill Medicare or Medicaid, but could bill all other payers. In reality no lab has ever lasted any time at all without a Certificate of Compliance. Thus I use the term "regulatory closure" as synonymous with revocation of the Certificate of Compliance.

I am aware of regulatory closure of only one lab in my 23 years experience in Pathology and Lab Medicine. It was a small clinic lab located about 125 miles from the municipality where I was living at the time. This lab was supposedly caught "sink testing". Sink testing is a type of fraud whereby the specimen is not tested; the specimen is discarded down a sink (hence the term "sink testing"), and a fraudulent lab report is generated. This fraudulent lab report typically indicates the patient has a normal test result, since normal lab results get little suspicion from the clinician.

This lab got caught because it was generating reports whereby the time of the reporting was before the time of collection. An astute clinician noticed this and made a complaint to the CMS. The CMS inspector came unannounced to this lab, and found that the lab did not have reagents or equipment to do testing, but had still turned out test results earlier on the day of inspection. The regulatory closure for this lab was immediate and happened on the spot when the sink testing was discovered.

To summarize, the possible outcomes of a CMS inspection are:

1. No citations. A Certificate of Compliance is issued without having to fill out form 2567
2. Few minor citations. The lab fills out form 2567 and it is accepted without revisions
3. Several minor citations. The form 2657 is accepted after one or more revisions
4. Significant citations. The lab is required to submit a Plan of Correction (PoC)
5. CMS makes a directed PoC for the lab
6. Severe citations. The lab is required to submit a Credible Allegation of Compliance (CAoC)
7. PoC or CAoC with one or more re-inspections.
8. Regulatory closure. (i.e. revocation of the CMS Certificate of Compliance).

In my experience, more than two rounds of modifying the form 2567 responses is unusual, having to file a Plan of Correction is rare and re-inspections are very rare. After your responses are accepted, you will get your notice of renewal from the CMS. This is followed by a bill. After you have paid the bill to CMS they will send your Certificate of Compliance.

The deemed status inspecting agencies use other accrediting documents such as a CAP Certificate of Accreditation. Irregardless of the inspecting agency, the certificate is good for two years from the date of issue. Your next regularly scheduled inspection will be in 2 years time. You can be inspected sooner than that if the inspecting agency receives one or more complaints about your lab.

If CMS can't complete an inspection by the time your existing Certificate of Compliance expires, they will grant an administrative extension of the old certificate. The CMS has limited numbers of inspectors, and has difficulty making travel arrangements to the most remote areas. In my experience working in remote areas, the biannual inspections can occur months after the old Certificate of Compliance has expired necessitating multiple administrative extensions of the old certificate. Once the biannual inspection is completed, the next Certificate of Compliance is set to expire 2 years after the old certificate had expired. The same problem does not usually occur in the continental US.

D. Testing your abilities to make a Plan of Correction

As a Lab Director writing Plans of Correction is an important part of your work. I will conclude this chapter with two Plan of Correction writing tests. The first **TEST** is a portion of the CMS form 2567 from my most recent inspection:

D5551	493.1271(a)(1)(f) IMMUNOHEMATOLOGY	D5551
540H 550H	The laboratory must perform ABO grouping, D(Rho) typing, unexpected antibody detection, antibody identification, and compatibility testing by following the manufacturer's instructions, if provided, and as applicable, 21 CFR 606.151(a) through (e). The laboratory must determine ABO group by concurrently testing unknown red cells with, at a minimum, anti-A and anti-B grouping reagents. For confirmation of ABO group, the unknown serum must be tested with known A1 and B red cells. The laboratory must determine the D(Rho) type by testing unknown red cells with anti-D (anti-Rho) blood typing reagent. The laboratory must document all control procedures performed, as specified in this section.	

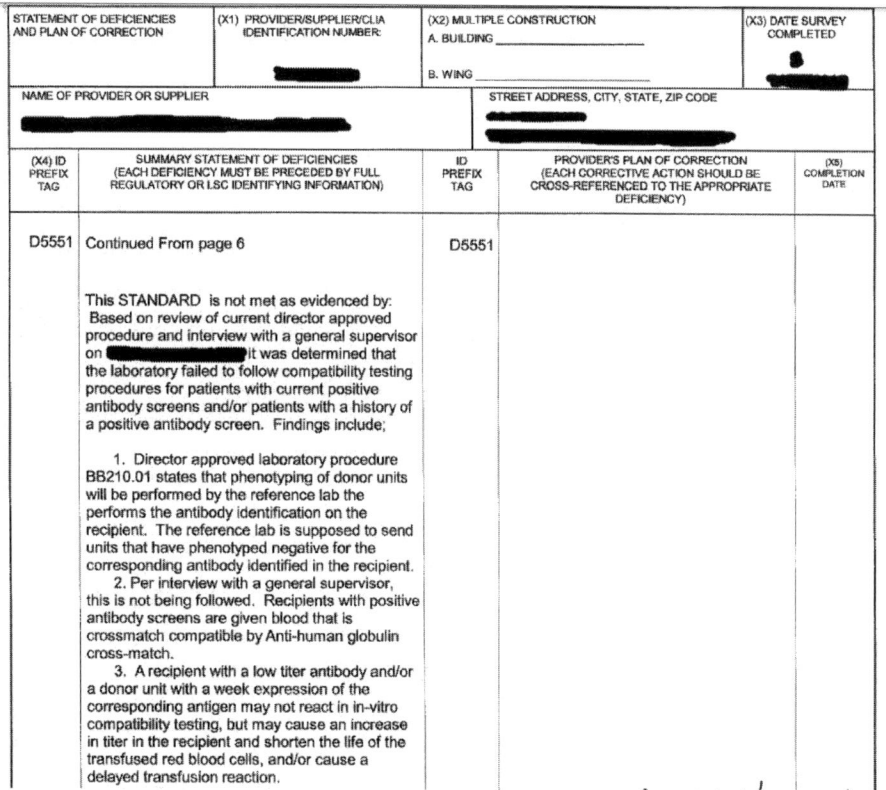

The Blood Bank has been cited for transfusing crossmatched blood to patients with unexpected antibodies without typing the donor units for the corresponding antigen. This is a standard level citation which could affect patient care.

The circumstances surrounding this citation are as follows. This is a small hospital lab Blood Bank with a relatively low volume, about 100 units transfused a month. There are about 6 patients a year with unexpected antibodies. The workup for the unexpected antibodies is sent out to the regional Blood Bank. If a request is made to transfuse a patient with an unexpected antibody, the small hospital Blood Bank is supposed to call the regional Blood Bank and ask them to send donor units negative for the corresponding antigen, and do the crossmatch using the specimen sent for antibody identification.

In reality what was happening is that the doctors involved would not wait for the antigen negative unit to come from the regional Blood Bank. The doctors were demanding immediate transfusion, and signing the emergency release forms to release crossmatched donor units from the local Blood Bank that had not been antigen typed. The donor unit antigen typing was not done after the fact. How would you respond to this citation?

The **ANSWER** to the citation could take one of two possible forms. First, enforce a rule that transfusion for patients with an unexpected antibody has to wait for the antigen negative blood to arrive from the regional Blood Bank. Second, start doing the donor unit antigen typing on-site.

This particular small hospital Blood Bank was very remote from the regional Blood Bank such that it would take 2 days or more for any units to arrive after being requested. Thus the first choice is not an option. Pick the second choice, starting antigen typing on-site.

In this case, the decision was made to continue sending the antibody identification to the regional Blood Bank. Once the results were received from the regional Blood Bank, the small hospital Blood Bank would be able to type donor units for the corresponding antigen.

Next, review the past 2 years of unexpected antibody data. The unexpected antibodies at this Blood bank were all from the Rh, Duffy, Kell, Kidd and Lewis systems. Request quotes for those antisera from your vendors. After the vendors respond write a Purchase Order to the vendor with the lowest-cost quote for the antisera. Make sure the antisera has the longest shelf life possible. You will be doing this typing only 6 times a year, and hardly using any of the antisera. The majority of what you order will expire.

Next write a procedure for the antigen typing. This is a common Blood Bank procedure and can be downloaded from the internet. Call a meeting of all the Blood Bank techs to inform them of the new procedure and if necessary show them how to do the procedure. Make sure they are aware that all patients with unexpected antibodies are to receive crossmatched donor units typed as negative for the corresponding antigen.

While reviewing the prior 2 years of unexpected antibody data from the files, there were 12 patients identified with unexpected antibodies. Most of them were pre-natal screens, and not transfused. Only 2 patients with unexpected antibodies were transfused. Pull the charts for those two patients, and review the charts to make sure there was no evidence of a hemolytic transfusion reaction.

You only need to review the past 2 years of data. Anything prior to that would predate the prior routine CMS inspection. You are only responsible for events occurring since the most recent routine CMS inspection 2 years ago.

Once you have that work done, you can write the Plan of Correction. Here is my Plan of Correction for the citation given above:

D5551) The lab has ordered antisera for typing of the relevant minor red blood cell antigens. A procedure has been written for typing of donor units for the minor red blood cell antigens. All Blood Bank staff have been informed of the new procedure, and the requirement to type donor units before crossmatching to a patient with known unexpected antibody or history of unexpected antibody at Blood Bank. The Blood Bank files have been reviewed for the past 2 years. There were 2 patients with a positive antibody screen or history of a positive antibody screen that received crossmatched blood without donor antigen typing. Review of the charts for these 2 patients reveals no evidence of harm to the patient. There were no hemolytic transfusion reactions.

This was typed into the right-hand column of form 2567, and sent in to the CMS along with copies of the vendor quote and Purchase Order for the antisera, and the procedure for antigen typing. The CMS accepted this response on the first try, without requiring any reworking.

If you are going to send your worksheets in to the CMS, be very careful to black out the patient names or other patient identifiers. Failure to black out patient information on documents sent in to the CMS is a HIPPA violation, and will get you into deeper trouble than the original citation.

The second Plan of Correction writing **TEST** is the second of the citations on my most recent CMS inspection.

D5411 320M	This STANDARD is not met as evidenced by:
	493.1252(a) TEST SYSTEMS, EQUIPMENT, INSTRUMENTS, REAGENT
	
	Test systems must be selected by the laboratory. The testing must be performed following the manufacturer's instructions and in a manner that provides test results within the laboratory's stated performance specifications for each test system as determined under §493.1253.
	
	This STANDARD is not met as evidenced by: Based on observation and interview with testing personnel on ▓▓▓▓▓▓▓▓▓ it was determined that the laboratory failed to have in place the appropriate procedure for the urinalysis methodology being used at the time of the survey. Findings included:
	
	   1. The manufacturer's package insert being used as the urinalysis dip-stick (macroscopic analysis) procedure was for Siemens Multistix.
	   2. The manufacturer's dip-stick in use at the time of the survey was Accutest URS10.
	   3. Testing personnel confirmed that there was no procedure in place for the manufacturer Accutest URS10.
		D5411

This involves the procedure for dipstick urinalysis. The vendor supplying lab had switched dipsticks from one manufacturer to another. The testing was the same, the interpretation was the same, everything about these dipsticks was the same except for the name on the container. Since everything about these dipsticks is identical I am assuming one is the generic and the other is the brand name for the same dipstick. However the name on the container changed. My lab had the name of the old manufacturer written into the procedure manual. The inspector caught this and gave us the citation above. How would you handle this?

ANSWER: This is a trick question. Dipstick urinalysis is a waived test. Waived tests do not need a procedure manual. All that is required for a waived test is that the manufacturer's package insert has to be available at the place and time of testing. The dipsticks in question arrived from the manufacturer with the package insert stuffed into the same cardboard tube as the dipsticks. The package insert was still present in the same tube as the dipsticks at the time of the CMS inspection. Thus we should never have been cited.

CMS inspectors are human, they make mistakes just like everybody else. My lab does testing of all three complexity levels: waived testing, moderate complexity testing and high complexity testing. Even though the urine dipsticks sit right next to high complexity testing equipment, urine dipstick is still a waived test. The CMS inspector got confused, and mistook dipstick urinalysis for a higher complexity test or otherwise would not have written us the citation above.

The question is how to respond to this mistaken citation. If you confront the CMS inspector head on, about 90% of the time they will admit they made a mistake and back down. The rest of the time, you will have just made an enemy that you can't afford to make. Thus in this situation, I played along, and make a corrective action as if urine dipstick is a moderate complexity test which it is not, it is a waived test.

Here is my approach to the Plan of Correction. The citation is a standard level citation. The two different tests have the same interpretation meaning that lab could not have turned out erroneous results for urine dipstick. Hence there is no need to track down patient charts. I added the name of the new manufacturer into the dipstick urinalysis procedure, signed and dated this change to the procedure manual. I did not strike the name of the old manufacturer from the procedure manual, in case the vendor ever switched us back to the old manufacturer. I added the package insert into the procedure manual, and I wrote the following for the Plan of Correction:

D5411) The urinalysis manual has been updated to reflect that either Accutest URS10 or Siemens Multistix may be used. The package insert for Accutest URS10 has been added to the procedure manual. The method of testing and interpretation are the same for both types of urine dipstick such that there was no risk of patient harm.

The Plan of Correction was typed into the right hand column of form 2567 and sent in to CMS. The CMS inspector accepted it the first try without requiring modifications. The entire time, the inspector never realized her mistake of requiring a procedure manual for a waived test.

It is possible to protest any of your citations. The only time I will protest a mistaken citation is if the Plan of Correction would entail significant outlays such as new equipment or new hires. The above Plan of Correction required writing in the procedure manual, and putting the package insert in the procedure manual. The package insert would have been discarded anyhow when the product was used up. Thus it did not cost anything to play along and make a Plan of Correction for this mistaken citation.

Vendor substitutions of one product for another happen occasionally. It usually means that the vendor was unable to obtain the exact same product you asked for. The vendor is supposed to ask permission from your lab beforehand for the switch. In this case, the vendor did not ask lab for permission to switch, and we found out when we got cited by the CMS. This should prompt a stern phone call to that vendor to remind them they are required to ask permission for a switch. This is also a good example of why you don't want to write the manufacturer's name into a procedure unless you have to.

Chapter 22 – Regulatory scrutiny syndrome

As a Lab Director, it is important that you keep you lab up to standards to the extent possible. I have noticed that once a lab has a bad inspection, the next time the inspectors come, they conduct a much more thorough inspection. This has the potential to put a lab on a downhill course that I refer to as "Regulatory Scrutiny Syndrome".

In the typical small hospital lab inspection CMS sends one inspector for one day. There is no way that one person can look over all the lab's documents in one day. In the typical small hospital lab, there are multiple sections (Blood Bank, hematology, chemistry, etc.). Each section will have hundreds of pages of procedure manuals. The quality assurance and proficiency testing may also run into the hundreds of pages for each section. Even a small hospital lab will have thousands of pages of documents. The inspector will only have time to look at a small sampling of the documents subject to review, due to the time constraints of the inspection.

If the inspector finds something seriously wrong, the findings will be documented. The next time this lab is inspected, it is likely there will be more than one inspector coming, and these inspectors are likely to stay for more than one day.

The typical small hospital lab is likely to have a few skeletons in the closet. Maybe a failed proficiency test but not two consecutive. Maybe several procedures are not well written, etc. This will likely not be noticed by one inspector on a one day inspection. However a team of inspectors given multiple days to inspect are not as subject to time constraints and can look at much more.

This team of inspectors is likely to find a great deal more wrong with the lab than was found at the initial inspection. The lab gets worse citations in the second inspection, and any subsequent inspection will involve even more inspectors staying for even more time and doing an even more thorough inspection.

In this manner, the lab ends up in a self-reinforcing cycle of more regulatory scrutiny leading to more problems found leading to even more regulatory scrutiny. I refer to this as Regulatory Scrutiny Syndrome. This is likely what happened to the municipal hospital that hired me in August, 2013 to "turnaround" its lab.

Once a lab starts on this downhill course it is very hard to pull up from this. In my experience it is more difficult to fix a lab with major problems than it is to start a whole new lab. In many cases it is less expensive to start a whole new lab than to fix up a lab with problems. Thus, many labs going down this slippery slope will voluntarily close down and cease to exist as a going concern. As a Lab Director, it is imperative that you should keep your lab up to standards at all times to the extent possible. You do not want to go down this slippery slope; it will lead to very unpleasant places.

A good part of my 23 years in Pathology and Lab Medicine has been spent at two municipal hospitals that were both struggling financially. In the first of these the supply and reagent shortages caused repeated citations on the inspections. It was a struggle to keep the lab up to par. One becomes very proficient at writing corrective actions when one works at such a hospital.

The second municipal hospital I worked at hired me in August, 2013 to "turnaround" a lab that had numerous citations for multiple problems. This lab had a PoC in place with CMS and 2 re-inspections following its August, 2012 regular inspection. The turnaround was completed quickly. By the time of the December, 2013 re-inspection all the citations from the prior inspection were corrected and only 2 additional minor citations were uncovered.

In my experience it is possible for a lab to pull back from the brink up until it gets regulatory closure. The second municipal hospital lab referenced above was very close to regulatory closure when I was hired.

As a Lab Director, lab "turnaround" is a dangerous profession. You are being hired by a lab that has a good chance of voluntarily closing down in the near term. Even worse, the federal government has a rule on the book, the reference is 42 U.S.C. § 263a(i)(3), stating that the Lab Director of any lab that has regulatory closure will not be allowed to own or operate a lab for the following 2 years.

If you are Lab Director of a lab that has regulatory closure, your name will go onto Medicare's "blacklist" of banned providers. CMS refers to this as the Medicare Exclusion Database (MED). Although it is supposed to be for only 2 years, once that 2 years is up you will have a difficult time getting your name off of the Medicare "blacklist" of banned providers.

I have spent a good part of my career as a lab "turnaround" specialist. In that time, I have been successful in pulling labs back from the brink. None of the labs I have directed has had regulatory closure. Thus, I have never been on the "banned" list.

The only Lab Director I know of that has been on the "banned" list is the director for the lab doing sink testing referenced above. That Lab Director never worked again in the field, in effect forced into retirement by the closure of his lab and by the Medicare ban which prevented him from getting work elsewhere. It took him an extended length of time for him to get his name off of the "banned" list. Even after he was off the "banned" list no one would hire him. The "banned" list acts as a de facto "blacklist" whereby no one in the field will ever hire anyone that has ever been on the "banned" list.

If you are considering working as a Lab Director at a lab with problems, speak privately with the CMS inspectors assigned to that lab. If the Lab Director position has been vacant for some time, as it tends to be at a deeply troubled lab, the CMS inspectors will be glad to see you come. Their job is to regulate labs; and they don't like having to shut labs down. Ask the CMS inspectors if the CMS intends to carry out regulatory closure on that lab. Ask for an unwritten agreement that if you take the position, they would inform you if regulatory closure ever becomes imminent for that lab. If regulatory closure becomes inevitable, resign from that Lab Directorship prior to the closure of the lab. You want to avoid the Medicare "blacklist" as it tends to be a career ender.

Chapter 23 – How to avoid HIPAA pitfalls

The Health Insurance Portability and Accountability Act of 1996 (known in the business as "HIPAA") regulates the release of Protected Health Information (PHI). PHI is defined as any individually identifiable health information. Using this definition, all lab results are PHI.

PHI can only be released in the following situations: to facilitate treatment, payment or health care operations, when consent has been granted by a patient, as required by law (i.e. under subpoena), when required for law enforcement, disclosure of communicable disease to the Public Health Department, research, government functions including disclosure of prisoner's lab results to a correctional facility, disclosure to the military, workers' compensation, etc.

HIPAA requires the hospital to take a number of actions such as designating a Privacy Official, training the workforce on HIPAA compliance, documenting the training, making a notice of privacy practices and giving the notice to all patients, making sure all policies and procedures comply with HIPAA, etc.

The hospital takes care of almost everything on this list. The lab HIPAA training and documentation of training are typically done by the hospital's HIPAA office, not the lab. The typical hospital lab is only responsible for making sure its policies and procedures are HIPAA compliant, and that lab staff comply with HIPAA.

With HIPAA there are basically only two types of mistakes you can make. First, you can give out PHI when you should not have. Second, you can withhold PHI when you should have given it out.

In my experience, labs are very tight-lipped. I have never seen a lab make the mistake of giving out PHI when it should not have. I have seen a number of instances of labs failing to give out PHI when they should have.

Failure to appropriately release PHI typically results from a request by an unknown doctor in an unknown city asking for one patient's lab results. Many labs will require a consent form signed by the patient, and will refuse to give out the information until a consent form signed by the patient is FAXed back. Under HIPAA, all the lab has to do is verify the requesting doctor is legitimate and is treating the patient in question, and then the test results can be given out.

All PHI except for lab results can be requested by the patient under HIPAA. At present HIPAA makes an exception for lab results and CLIA prohibits labs from giving test results directly to the patient. There are some proposed changes to both CLIA and HIPPA that would correct this situation, but at present a lab cannot give results directly to the patient.

As a result, most hospital labs can handle every permutation of lab result request except for a patient walking into lab and demanding his or her own lab results. In my experience, this happens a number of times a year, particularly when a patient is traveling to see a specialist in a larger city. The patient has to go to the airport for the next flight out, and doesn't have time to go back to the doctor's office to get the lab results from the doctor.

The way I handle this situation is as follows. I print a copy of the patient's test results, and walk with the patient down to the hospital's Medical Records Department. Under HIPAA the Lab is allowed to release lab results to the hospital's Medical Records Department. I hand off the lab results to the person at the front desk of the Medical Records Department. The Medical Records Department is allowed under HIPAA to release the results to the patient. The Medical Records Department checks the patient's ID, gives the printout to the patient, and makes the patient sign for the release of his or her own lab results.

Chapter 24 – How to interact with the legal profession

As a Lab Director there are two ways you could get called into court. The first is that your lab could be sued over test results produced in your lab. This would be a malpractice suit, and you would be a party to the suit. This has never happened in my experience. In my 23 years in Pathology and Lab Medicine, no lab I have ever worked for has ever been sued over the lab results generated. Nor to the best of my knowledge has any other lab in any municipality where I have ever lived. I assume that the process would be similar to that described below, with the exception that you are a party to the suit, not a disinterested bystander.

Much more commonly, you will be called as an expert witness to testify in a case whereby you are not a party to the lawsuit, but the testing was done in your lab. The most common situations are paternity testing and testing for Driving Under the Influence (DUI). In these cases you are not a party to the lawsuit. In a DUI trial the parties to the lawsuit are the DUI driver (the Defendant) and the Attorney General's (AG's) Office (i.e. the Prosecutor). You are a disinterested party called in to testify on questions related to the alcohol testing done in your laboratory.

In my career I have worked at two municipal hospitals. In both municipalities, the procedure for DUI states that if a suspicious driver is stopped, the police do a field sobriety test and/or breath test. If the driver fails either or both tests, the driver is taken to the municipal hospital lab for the blood test. The testing is done in Lab. The entire DUI case turns on the outcome of this testing, and you will occasionally be called into court to testify that the Lab did the testing properly. This happens about once every year or two at the typical municipal hospital.

If you receive this call of duty from the AG's Office it will be in the form of a subpoena. This is literally an invitation you can't refuse. If you fail to show up for this scheduled court appearance you could be jailed. The subpoena will show up in the form of a Sheriff coming into the lab and asking for you by name. Try not to have a heart attack when a uniformed law enforcement officer shows up in lab and asks for you by name. The law enforcement officer will hand you the subpoena and ask you to sign for receipt.

Most hospitals' procedure manuals require that you inform the hospital legal department and/or risk manager immediately if you receive a subpoena. Call them and inform them of the subpoena. The hospital's legal department and/or risk manager should be able to give you all the advice you need.

Like all patient test results, alcohol results are covered by HIPAA and are confidential. In this case, you have a legal mandate in the form of a subpoena requesting the information. HIPAA allows for disclosure of the confidential information in this circumstance. Be careful to only disclose the information to the Prosecutor, Defendant's Attorney or any court official with a reasonable need to know. Do not disclose the alcohol results to anyone that does not need to know as part of the court proceeding.

Most hospital administrative manuals state that you will need the permission of the hospital's legal department and/or risk manager to release any test results outside the hospital. In almost all circumstances they will approve of the release of information requested by the subpoena. If they disapprove, they will send the hospital's attorney into court to try to "quash" the subpoena.

Next, call the Prosecutor whose name appears on the subpoena. Ask the Prosecutor the details of the case such as the date of the testing and name of the Defendant. Look up the testing records for that Defendant, and the relevant QC. In particular make sure the controls were in for the alcohol testing on that day of testing. Make a note of the dates of calibration immediately prior to and after the Defendant's testing.

Make copies of the alcohol test results and chain of custody form. Once you have the hospital's permission for external release of this information, provide the copies to the Prosecutor and Defendant's Attorney. You will be asked to provide your resume or Curriculum Vita (CV) to both the Prosecutor and the Defendant's Attorney.

Make sure that your CV lists all your qualifications. This includes not only Anatomic Pathology and Clinical Pathology Board Certification (if applicable), but also sub-specialty training, other training, publications, books written, etc. The Prosecutor and Defendant's Attorney will review your CV. The Prosecutor will almost never object to your credentials. If you are Board Certified, the Defendant's Attorney will not likely question your credentials.

The Defendant's Attorney would rather not have you at the trail, and rarely will question your credentials in the long-shot hope of getting you disqualified as an expert witness. If the Defendant's Attorney objects to your credentials, your credentials will be presented to the Judge before the trail starts. The Prosecutor will inform the Judge that you are Board Certified, and this is the highest training possible in a clinical lab. The Judge will almost certainly admit you as an expert witness.

The decision on admitting you to court as an expert witness has to be made before the trail starts. You will be informed of this decision in advance of the trail. There should be no objections to your credentials during the trail. As noted below, the Defendant's Attorney may question your credentials at the trial, but can't make an outright objection to your credentials at the trial since this matter has been settled in advance of the trial.

The majority of the time there will be no objections to your credentials. If the Defendant's Attorney does not object to your credentials before the trail starts, the Defendant's Attorney has accepted you as an expert witness.

As an expert witness you should be available to both the Prosecutor and the Defendant's Attorney. Answer phone calls and meet with either side as requested. You can set the schedule to your own convenience. You do not need to have the Prosecutor on the phone line when talking with the Defendant's Attorney, and vice versa. You do not need to have the Prosecutor present to meet with the Defendant's Attorney, and vice versa. You are an independent expert, not beholden to either side of the trail.

It is not uncommon to get phone calls from both the Defendant's Attorney and Prosecutor before the case comes to trial. The lawyers won't be very familiar with lab testing and will phrase the questions in general terms: "Was the lab testing good?" "Was there a problem with the lab testing?".

You may or may not be called for depositions. A deposition is a formal meeting between the Prosecutor and the Defendant's Attorney. If you are called into a deposition you will be given the oath. Be very careful to answer truthfully while under oath. The deposition will be recorded and later transcribed.

By the time of the deposition, both the Prosecutor and the Defendant's Attorney should have copies of the chain of custody form. They are usually satisfied with the chain of custody form, and you will not be questioned much on it. You will be asked a few general questions about the testing for that particular DUI case. Was the testing good? Was there a problem with the testing?

Some time later, you may be asked to sign a transcript of the deposition. Be careful to check the transcript very carefully for transcription errors. You can't change your testimony after the fact. However, there are usually transcription errors to correct, since the transcriptionist is usually a legal secretary with little to no medical knowledge.

If it is a simple DUI with no injuries, it will likely get settled by plea bargain and you won't be called for depositions or called into court. If the case is a vehicular homicide with DUI there is less chance of a plea bargain and it is much more likely you will be called for depositions and the case will go to trial. A case of DUI with injuries but no fatalities falls somewhere in between. If the case goes to court, you will be notified of the court date.

You will need to take one or more days off from work to do the court testifying. In both municipal hospitals I worked at this was allowed to be administrative leave with pay. Since the request was coming from a different agency of the same municipality, the hospital could not ask you to use your own annual leave (vacation time) to do the testifying.

You have to sit in court all day waiting for your turn to testify. Since the Prosecutor does not know the exact order of the cases in advance, you have to come early and wait all day for the case to come up.

No talking is permitted in the seating area inside the courtroom. Everyone has to turn off their cellphones and pagers. You have to go outside to talk. As a result, the courtroom will be quieter than any library you have ever been in. The room is completely silent except for the Judge, lawyers and the defendants quietly talking at the front of this large room. It can be a struggle to stay awake all day under these conditions. It is embarrassing to have your name called and be caught sleeping in the seating area of the courtroom.

Bring a copy of all relevant paperwork with you to the trial. Read it all so as to prepare yourself for the testimony. If there have been depositions, read the transcripts from end to end. This will help you to remember all the details. It will also make good reading material as you struggle to stay awake all day in this silent room.

Eventually, the case in question comes before the court and then your name is called as an expert witness. You will be directed to the witness stand. It is really a chair, not a stand, you will be seated in front of the jury during your testimony. Next, they administer the oath. You will be told to place one hand on a bible and will be asked something to the effect "Do you swear to tell the truth, the whole truth, and nothing but the truth?". The only acceptable answer is "I do".

Next, you are introduced to the jury as an expert witness. There may be a short recitation of your credentials. Your testimony begins with the Prosecutor asking you to present your findings. This is known as the direct examination. When and where was the testing done? What was the outcome of the test?

Answer the questions truthfully and to the best of your abilities. Speak clearly. Some courts do not have a microphone in which case you have to speak loudly enough to be heard in the furthest back row of the courtroom. Keep all explanations in layman's terms. In most jurisdictions, the minimum qualification for a juror is high school graduation or equivalent. Your explanations should be simple enough for a high school senior to understand. Do not give extraneous information unrelated to the question that was asked. If a fact is important, one side or the other will eventually ask you about it.

After the Prosecutor is done questioning you, the Defendant's Attorney will question you. This is known as the cross-examination. The Defendant's Attorney will try to cast doubt on the case in any way possible. The evidence is stacked against the Defendant, otherwise the case would not have been prosecuted. The Defendant's Attorney knows that he is playing a losing hand, and is usually desperate to win the case any way possible.

Be prepared that the Defendant's Attorney will try to attack your credentials as an expert witness. You will be peppered with questions like "What are you qualifications? ", "Are you sure you're qualified to be an expert witness?", "How long have you been an expert witness?"

My assessment: If you are Board Certified in Clinical Pathology, that is all you need. You are an expert in lab testing, and the case turns on the lab test for alcohol. Given the context of this case you really are an expert, even if this is the first time you have served as an expert witness.

Do not take this questioning by the Defendant's Attorney personally. The Defendant's Attorney is just doing his or her job, trying every maneuver possible to get the Defendant acquitted. At this stage of the questioning, the important point is to stay calm and stay focused on the testimony at hand. Do not get into an argument with the Defendant's Attorney. If you get into an argument while on the witness stand, it will only serve to discredit you, which will play into the hands of the Defendant's Attorney. Stay focused on the testimony at hand and do not lose your concentration.

Next the Defendant's Attorney will try to question the testing: "Are you really sure the test is positive?", "How do you determine a positive test in your lab"?, "Did your lab follow the correct chain of custody?"

My assessment: Answer the questions honestly and to the best of your abilities. Remember that you are under oath. If you get caught lying under oath, the consequences would be devastating to your career. In most cases the answers are straightforward "Yes, the test is positive," "Yes, we followed the correct chain of custody".

If there was a problem with the test, such as the controls were out on that day of testing, you have to inform the court at this point. Since you had previously been on the phone or in depositions with both the Defendant's Attorney and the Prosecutor, there should be no surprises in your testimony.

If you say something different in the trail compared to the prior depositions, phone calls, etc. you should explain why you changed your mind. If there are discrepancies between your prior testimony and the testimony on the day of trial, the Defendant's Attorney will notice and point out every last discrepancy to the jury. The Defendant's Attorney is looking to discredit you. If you repeatedly change your mind, you will be helping the Defendant's Attorney to discredit you.

Keep in mind that you are an expert in Lab only. The Defendant's Attorney may ask you questions that are beyond your area of expertise. If this happens do not answer the question and state that your area of expertise is limited to Lab. If the Defendant's Attorney asks inappropriate questions or makes a personal attack such as "you are unqualified" the Prosecutor will object.

If you do not know the answer to any question, state that you do not know. It is very unlikely for the Prosecutor to ask you a question you can't answer. The Prosecutor needs your testimony to help win the case. Thus the Prosecutor is not looking to discredit you. The Defendant's Attorney is more likely to ask a question that you are unable to answer. The Defendant's Attorney is hoping that you will answer a question beyond your area of expertise, or beyond your possible range of knowledge. If you fall into this trap, the Defendant's Attorney will discredit you with the intent of discrediting your testimony.

After the Defendant's Attorney is done questioning you the court is then open to all questions. This is basically a free-for-all whereby both the Prosecutor and the Defendant's Attorney can ask you anything they want. Both attorneys are under pressure and making questions on-the-fly at this point. Be prepared for some bizarre questions, especially from the Defendant's Attorney. Take your time answering the questions, and avoid feeling pressured to answer quickly. If one side asks an inappropriate question, the other side will object.

After this round of questioning is done you will be excused from the witness stand. The typical DUI trial lasts only a day or two. You will not be informed of the results (conviction, acquittal or last-minute plea bargain). If you are curious you can find out by calling the Prosecutor's Office a few days later.

I am a golfer and from time to time meet some of the Prosecutors from the AG's office while golfing. As we sit in the clubhouse after the golf game we chat about topical matters, I bring up the issue of DUI. They tell me that the plea bargain offered for First Offense DUI is so lenient you have to be crazy to turn down the offer. Very few people contest a First Offense DUI. That is why I am only called in once every year or two to testify. Very few people get a Second Offense DUI or higher number DUI offense. Those that do have a serious drug and/or alcohol problem, and for them the jail time is really drug/alcohol rehab time.

The process for testifying in a paternity testing case is similar to the DUI cases described above. In my 23 years in Pathology and Lab Medicine I have been called to testify in paternity testing cases 4 times. This comes out to once in about 5 years.

In a paternity testing case the alleged father is the Defendant and the municipal Department of Social Services (or similar agency) is the Plaintiff. The case is a civil lawsuit, not a criminal trial.

Here is a brief summary of the process. A child is born to an unmarried woman. If the paternity is undisputed the mother and father sign the birth certificate. If the paternity is disputed the mother contacts the municipal agency that handles child support. In most municipalities this is known as the Department of Social Services. Other possible names include the Department of Human Services, Local Child Support Agency, etc.

The Department of Social Services serves papers on the alleged father. The alleged father will need to hire an attorney at this point. The case will go to court and the Judge will issue a court order requiring paternity testing.

Specimens must be collected from the alleged father, the mother and child for testing. For lab testing purposes, the court order is accepted as equivalent to a Physician's orders for testing. The specimens are usually collected at the local municipal hospital lab and sent to a reference lab for testing. The results come back to the municipal hospital lab and are transmitted to the court

If your lab does paternity testing, or collects the specimens for paternity testing, it is imperative that your lab should require two valid photo IDs of the alleged father that comes in for testing. Your lab should make copies of the photo IDs presented by the alleged father at the time of specimen collection.

Paternity testing is currently done by genetic testing. Testing by blood groups is obsolete. The genetic testing used in this type of case is much more complicated than the alcohol testing in a DUI case. Neither the Plaintiff's Attorney nor the Defendant's Attorney will have much understanding of the testing and will need you to explain the testing to them, the jurors and the Judge.

The proceedings follow the same layout as for the DUI trial described above. You will receive a subpoena. Drop a copy of the subpoena with the hospital's legal counsel and/or risk manager. The subpoena will likely be followed by one or more phone calls from the Plaintiff's Attorney and Defendant's Attorney. You may or may not be called in for depositions.

Make additional copies of the two valid photo IDs that the alleged father had produced to your lab on the day of testing. These copies should be provided to both the Plaintiff's Attorney and the Defendant's Attorney.

In a paternity testing case, the Defendant's Attorney will oftentimes question whether you have done the paternity testing on the right person. The Defendant's Attorney may make the claim that someone else, not the alleged father, had come in for the testing. Hence the need for the two photo IDs of the person who showed up for paternity testing. Otherwise, the process is similar to the DUI cases described above.

Paternity cases are frequently settled prior to trial. If the genetic testing conclusively proves paternity, the Defendant will oftentimes acquiesce, and admit paternity. This obviates the need for a trial. If the case goes to trail, the procedure is the same for direct examination, cross-examination, and free-for-all questioning.

At the trial, you will be under oath. Answer the questions truthfully and to the best of your abilities. Keep all explanations in layman's terms. In most jurisdictions, the minimum qualification for a juror is high school graduation or equivalent. Your explanations should be simple enough for a high school senior to understand. Since the testing for a paternity case is more complex than the alcohol testing in a DUI case, it is much more difficult to explain this in simple layman's terms.

There is one final point to make. In both DUI cases and paternity testing cases the prosecuting attorney is an official of the municipality where you live. If you are Lab Director of the municipal hospital you too are an official of the same municipality. Even so, an expert witness is supposed to be an unbiased, disinterested party to the legal proceeding. Do not put any "spin" or bias on your testimony so as to favor the prosecution. Let the chips fall where they may.

Chapter 25 – How to be a waived test Lab Director and a PPM Lab Director

Under CLIA the Lab Director for waived testing can be any physician. Pathology training is only required for moderate and high complexity testing. Thus, the majority of this book has been directed to moderate and high complexity testing.

Waived testing is commonly referred to as "Point Of Care (POC) testing". I consider that to be a misnomer, and prefer the term "waived test". By definition a waived test is so simple that a high school graduate can do the test with little risk of making a mistake if the manufacturer's instructions are followed. The significance of the test is typically low, such that erroneous results are unlikely to make a difference in patient outcome.

CMS requires that any testing facility that does waived testing needs to have a Certificate of Waiver if it does not already have a Certificate of Compliance. In other words if you have an outpatient lab with no CMS certificates (i.e. not doing any tests at all) and you want to add waived testing you need a Certificate of Waiver from CMS. If you are already doing moderate and/or high complexity testing and have a Certificate of Compliance, you do not need an additional certificate from CMS in order to add waived testing.

If you need a Certificate of Waiver, you must apply for and receive it before starting the waived testing. When doing the testing you are obligated to follow the manufacturer's instructions. You are required to pay the fee for the Certificate of Waiver and required to notify the CMS within 30 days of any changes in ownership, name, location or Lab Director for the lab.

Other than the above requirements these tests are "waived" meaning that CMS waives all other testing requirements. You do not have to do calibration, calibration verification, determine Analytic Measurement Range (AMR), write a procedure manual, etc. You can assign high school graduates as testing personnel, the requirement for a lab tech degree is waived. There is no need for training and competency testing for the personnel doing the test; these are waived as well.

The manufacturer's instructions typically require you to run three levels of control on the day of testing. Even though CLIA doesn't require controls, you will still be running controls because CLIA requires you to follow the manufacturer's instructions.

There have been several instances in my career where I have been asked to take on the Lab Directorship for waived testing, since no one else wanted the Lab Directorship. For an example, a Family Practice doctor wanted to do waived fingerstick glucose and urine dipstick testing in his office. This Family Practice doctor felt completely out of place doing anything with lab testing. He felt that he has absolutely no knowledge or understanding of lab, and couldn't handle the Lab Directorship of waived testing. He had an Internist and two Pediatricians working for him in his small clinic, but none of them wanted the Lab Directorship or felt that they could handle it. I was called and asked to serve as Lab Director for this facility.

A waived testing Lab Directorship does not count towards the maximum of 5 Lab Directorships that CLIA allows. I took on the Lab Directorship of this waived testing, since no one else wanted it and the testing was felt to be essential to that particular outpatient clinic.

The application form was sent in to CMS, and they sent a bill and some associated paperwork. Once the bill was paid, the Certificate of Waiver came back a few weeks later. In my experience, CMS issuance of a Certificate of Waiver is a knee-jerk reflex whereby to the best of my knowledge they have never turned down an application for a Certificate of Waiver. As soon as you receive the Certificate of Waiver, you can begin testing.

As Lab Director for this lab, your responsibilities include making sure the staff follow the instructions, and making sure that they write the results for the controls in the control log. The first day testing is started, come out to the lab for a few hours at the start of business to show them how to operate the test equipment and how to write control results in a control log. Bring several blank copies of control log sheets with you when you come and drop these off with the outpatient clinic. Observe them doing the testing a few times to make sure they are following the instructions.

It should be made very clear to the testing personnel that they should never release test results if the controls are out. Instruct them that is the controls are out, they are to call the hospital lab for help, and someone will be dispatched to help them. In my experience, I have never seen a waived test repeatedly fail controls when the instructions are being followed.

If you receive this call of duty to come back to the small outpatient lab due to failed controls, it almost certainly means they are performing the test improperly. When you come, the main thing you will be looking for is whether they are following the instructions. Other possibilities include something wrong with the controls (outdated controls, hemolyzed controls, etc.). For disposable test kits, check the expiration date on the test kit. Check the storage conditions (too hot or cold) for the waived testing supplies and equipment. Glucose meters and other similar equipment can wear out over time, and may need to be maintenanced or replaced.

Once you have the waived testing up and running, it should not require more than about an hour a month of work on your part. I usually make the trip to these waived testing clinics on Saturday mornings. This is mainly because my hospital lab job requires me to be on site weekdays from 8AM to 5PM.

In your trips to the waived testing clinic you will mainly be checking that they are following the manufacturer's instructions, keeping the package insert readily available at the time and place of testing, running controls on each day of testing, maintaining the controls log, and all the controls are in. If they are doing testing daily they should become familiar with the testing procedure very quickly. If they are not doing the test very often, they may need an occasional refresher.

It is possible to intentionally modify an existing test, be it waived, moderate complexity or high complexity. Any test so modified automatically becomes a high complexity test. This would be particularly problematic at a waived testing site. The waived testing site is not doing any of the quality assurance work associated with high complexity testing. Thus, you must be very careful that no one at the waived testing site intentionally modifies the test.

My advice on this issue is that you should never intentionally modify a test, even a high complexity test in the main part of the hospital lab. If you do so, you will essentially become the manufacturer for your new test, responsible for all sorts of work such as making the Analytical Measurement Range (AMR), reference range, etc. Avoid modifying tests, unless you like to do a huge amount of work that isn't really necessary.

There is one big caveat here. You can add more waived testing onto a Certificate of Waiver but you cannot add moderate or high complexity testing. Some analyzers are capable of both waived testing and more complex testing. Be very careful when adding tests to these types of equipment.

For example an Abbot I-stat can do glucose and chemistries as a waived test. However, if you add on BNP to the same Abbot I-stat the BNP testing is moderate complexity. In other words this one piece of equipment will be doing testing of two different levels of complexity. If you do this, you will have exceeded the scope of the Certificate of Waiver. You now need a Certificate of Compliance for the moderate complexity testing being done on that same piece of equipment.

I have known at least one small clinic to get itself into trouble this way, by adding on testing that was beyond the scope of its Certificate of Waiver. If you are Lab Director of any lab doing moderate complexity testing and that lab only has a Certificate of Waiver you will be in deep trouble with the CMS inspectors when they find out about it. If you have a Lab Directorship at a small clinic doing waived testing, make sure it is very clear to them that they need your approval before adding any tests.

A waived testing lab is not subject to routine CMS inspections, but you have to allow the inspectors to come if they want to. In my experience, when the CMS inspectors are in town, they stick to the moderate and/or high complexity testing labs, and bypass all the small clinics with Certificates of Waiver. If they do stop by a waived testing site, the inspection typically lasts less than an hour. The CMS inspectors will check your control log for a few minutes, spend half an hour making sure that your staff are following the instructions properly, and then the inspectors move on.

When I first started in Pathology and Lab Medicine there were very few waived tests. At present, there is a long list of waived tests. In my opinion waived testing is taking over, and the future of lab testing seems to be heading towards all or nearly all waived testing.

In circumstances where I have to add a new test that cannot go onto existing equipment in my lab, I try to add a waived test if available, in preference to adding a moderate or high complexity test. Even though the hospital labs I run have Certificates of Compliance, I preferentially add waived tests since a waived test is so much easier to deal with from a regulatory perspective.

Provider Performed Microscopy (PPM) is much more common in the outpatient setting than in a hospital lab. CMS requires that any testing facility that does PPM needs to have a Certificate of PPM if it does not already have a Certificate of Compliance. In other words if you have an outpatient lab with a Certificate of Waiver (i.e. doing waived tests only) and you want to add PPM you need an additional certificate from CMS. If you are already doing moderate and/or high complexity testing and have a Certificate of Compliance, you do not need an additional certificate from CMS.

The Lab Director of a PPM lab can be a physician of any specialty, dentist or a midlevel practitioner (nurse midwife, nurse practitioner, or physician assistant) licensed in the State where the testing is done. In this regard, the standards are even lower than the standards for waived testing. However, CMS considers PPM to be a subset of moderate complexity testing.

The qualification for the testing personnel is the same as the qualification for the Lab Director (physician, dentist or midlevel practitioner licensed in the State where the testing is done). Hence, in every PPM test site I am aware of, the Lab Director is the same as the person that does the test.

The list of PPM tests is wet mounts, KOH preps, pinworm exams, fern test, post-coital direct qualitative examinations of mucous, urinalysis with microscopic exam with or without dipstick, fecal leukocyte examination, semen analysis and nasal smears for eosinophils.

The PPM test site must have a procedure manual. The PPM provider should not need training on how to do the test. If the provider has not had training during their education on how to do the test, the provider should not be doing the test.

Each PPM provider must have competency testing at least annually for each PPM procedure done by that provider. The competency testing is done in the same manner as for lab tech competency testing described in a prior chapter. The CMS rules for competency testing are the same for PPM providers as for lab techs. Proficiency testing is required for all PPM tests.

In this setting, controls consist of example positive and negative slides to compare the patient specimen to. Correlation would be possible by showing 20 unknown slides to different PPM providers and correlating the results. I have never seen correlation done for PPM testing.

The remainder of lab quality control is not applicable to PPM testing. There is no such thing as PPM calibration, verification of calibration, analytic measurement range, reportable range or linearity. The test consists of a provider looking down a microscope at a specimen that the provider has collected.

There is a normal range for each test (negative for pinworms, negative for nasal eosinophils, etc.). The concept of a critical result (panic value) is not applicable since the provider does not need to call himself or herself to inform himself or herself of the result.

I have never been called upon to be the Lab Director of a PPM testing site. I could do so if called upon, but that call of duty has never materialized.

Chapter 26 - How to start a new lab from nothing

There are two ways a large lab can start. It can grow from a small lab or it can be built as a large lab from the beginning.

In my 23 years experience in Pathology and Lab Medicine, I have only once helped in the founding of a large lab. This lab was built in a small municipality where I lived for several years. Here is the story.

Some years ago a pharmacist founded his own company, selling pharmaceuticals to the small to mid-size clinics in this small town. Although ostensibly a pharmaceutical company it was really more of a general medical merchandise store. This small town lacked medical suppliers, and the pharmacist-businessman stepped in to fill the vacuum. His company sold everything from orthotics to pharmaceuticals to waived testing kits.

The pharmacist-businessman was very experienced in pharmacy and CMS regulations pertaining to pharmacy. He was also surprisingly knowledgeable about Lab and CMS regulations pertaining to lab.

He had approached several small doctor's offices and clinics offering to supply them with all sorts of medical merchandise including waived testing kits. In some instances the doctors would say that they wanted waived tests, but they did not feel they could handle the Lab Directorship or the regulatory aspects of the testing.

The pharmacist-businessman made the following deal with the doctors. The pharmacist-businessman will fill out the CMS forms with the doctor's name as Lab Director for the waived testing. The CMS certificate will come with that doctor's name on it as the Lab Director. However, the pharmacist-businessman will do all the Lab Director work, to include educating the staff, checking the control logs for completeness, CLIA compliance, etc.

This arrangement is entirely legitimate. Under CLIA the Lab Director of waived testing labs can delegate the entirety of the Lab Directorship to someone else, and do no work whatsoever.

This pharmacist-businessman got about 20 clinics to sign up for his waived testing program. Before this waived testing program started, there was only one lab in this town. It was the local satellite lab of a Regional Reference Lab. The Regional Reference Lab was very unhappy when a competitor set up shop in a town that lab formerly had a monopoly on.

This pharmaceutical company was supplying waived testing kits, equipment and supplies for almost all testing that could be done as a waived test. This includes electrolytes, glucose, lipid panel, complete metabolic profile, etc.

However, there is no waived testing for CBCs. All CBC testing is moderate complexity. The pharmaceutical company would have to collect up all the CBC specimens and send them to the Regional Reference Lab they were in competition with. No businessman anywhere likes to send work to the competition; it means that you do not make money and your competition makes money instead.

This pharmacist-businessman decided that it would make good business sense to set up his own lab to do the CBC testing, instead of sending the CBCs to the competition. Since this is moderate complexity testing, he needed a Pathologist to be Lab Director.

At the time, I was the only civilian pathologist in this small town. When I received the call from this pharmacist-businessman, I told him that I was the Lab Director of the municipal hospital in this small town. I'd have to check if it would be a conflict of interest before taking the outside position on.

The municipal hospital only did inpatient testing. The municipality's procurement code was so convoluted that if outpatients wanted lab testing at the municipal hospital, they would have to fill out a great deal of paperwork before being drawn. The pharmacist-businessman's waived testing and the Regional Reference Lab both had a streamlined process of collecting specimens. No outpatient testing was going to the hospital.

The municipal hospital does not do outpatient testing, and the proposed outside lab will do no inpatient testing. Hence, they are not in competition. The municipal hospital lab isn't going to be doing any direct business with the proposed outside lab.

I spoke to the Municipal Hospital Administrator, relaying the request for me to help with setting up the outside lab. As far as I can tell, it is not conflicted with my job at the municipal hospital.

The Municipal Hospital Administrator said that I could take on the project provided that I was still committed to doing the municipal hospital work Monday to Friday 8AM to 5PM. The outside work could be done on weekends and/or after hours.

CLIA sets a limit of 5 lab directorships per person. I was not reaching my limit on lab directorships at this time, so this limit did not stand in my way of taking on another position.

I called back the pharmacist-businessman and told him that I can take the position, and help him set up CBC testing. The analyzer was put in a warehouse that also housed pharmaceuticals. I followed the procedure to install new equipment as outlined in a prior chapter. The pharmacist-businessman was responsible for putting in place the computer system, billing, reporting and administrative mechanisms for the new lab. He placed the advertisements for lab staff, and I evaluated the resumes.

Things went very well for this new lab. A year later, the pharmacist-businessman decided to add a chemistry analyzer to his lab. The cost of testing for chemistries is lower for moderate complexity than waived testing.

The throughput is much higher for moderate complexity chemistry testing. Some of the clinics that were doing the waived testing were having staffing problems, and didn't want to commit the staff time to waived testing. It is much faster to draw a tube of blood, and make someone else test it.

The year after the CBC analyzer went live, I helped put the chemistry analyzer into service. The following year, the pharmacist-businessman wanted to add microbiology testing in-house. He was sending all microbiology testing to his competitors, the Regional Reference Lab. As mentioned above, nobody likes to send paying work to the competition. Furthermore, by this time the relationship between the pharmacist-businessman and the Regional Reference Lab had soured, as I will detail in the next chapter.

The microbiology equipment needs to have a hood with exhaust. However, the lab was housed in a warehouse that was primarily intended for pharmaceuticals. The microbiology equipment could not be set up in that warehouse. If it was, the exhaust from the microbiology hood could contaminate the area where the pharmaceutical supply techs were working. The lab would have to be set up in a different building in order to accommodate the microbiology hood. Medical office building space was selected that had a ventilating system capable of accommodating the microbiology exhaust ducts.

This is an example of why you have to be careful when choosing new equipment to purchase. As I mentioned in the chapter on putting a new analyzer into commission, you have to be very careful that a new piece of equipment will fit into the space allotted and will not have any unusual requirements such as special water supply, special electricity supply, etc. that would exceed the resources available in the lab where the equipment is to be located.

In this case, the situation was unavoidable. It was not possible to put a microbiology hood into that pharmacy warehouse. Two years prior, when the CBC analyzer was put into that warehouse, nobody knew that the lab would be very successful and grow so rapidly. If anyone had foreseen that the lab would expand so rapidly, the CBC analyzer would have gotten its own office space, not a pharmacy warehouse.

The problem is that the CBC analyzers and chemistry analyzers would have to be physically moved from their current location. There is supposedly a small risk that moving equipment can damage it, or otherwise cause it to become inaccurate

The typical procedure used when moving a piece of equipment is to split 20 samples, run a split before the move and run a split after the move. Correlate the analyzer as it was at the old site to the analyzer as it is now at the new site. I would also recommend recalibrating and running calibration verification after the move.

Two years after its start this lab is offering CBCs, microbiology, and chemistry testing on site. Over the course of the next 3 years this lab would add coagulation testing, urinalysis, etc. on site so as to become more of a full service lab. It does not offer anatomic pathology or blood banking in-house. The volume of testing did not justify this.

This lab was built over the course of 5 years, constructed one analyzer at a time. I consider it one of my greatest accomplishments, almost as difficult as the 2013 "turnaround" of a troubled lab described in a prior chapter.

In my 23 years experience in Pathology and Lab Medicine I have only once seen an entirely new hospital built in the community where I lived. It was an 80 bed hospital. The construction of the lab was contracted out a firm in a large city.

From the time the structure topped out until the opening of the hospital was only 6 months. The process of building the new hospital's lab would be the same as that described above for the outpatient lab. The only difference would be that all the analyzers would be getting put into the same lab at the same time. Each analyzer would follow the procedure for putting a new analyzer into commission given in a chapter above.

There would likely be multiple Service Reps, Lab Directors and lab techs working as multiple teams with each team assigned to set up one or a few analyzers. There would likely be on overall Lab Director supervising the various teams setting up the analyzers. That overall Lab Director would have to pay particular attention to space constraints and time constraints given so much work being done in a limited area and limited time.

Chapter 27 – Lab Director ethics

As a Lab Director, you are expected to uphold the same code of ethics as any other Medical Doctor. The medical code of ethics dates back to Hippocrates and enumerates certain basic rights that patients have. Patients have a right to autonomy (the right to make their own decisions), beneficence (always act in the patient's best interest) and non-maleficence (avoid harm to the patient). The distribution of medical care must be fair and just.

Some lab organizations have created their own codes of ethics. These tend to stipulate additional requirements such as duty to the profession, duty to the community, commitment to excellence, dedication to competence, showing compassion and respect to the patient, continuing medical education, maintaining confidentiality, respect human rights, etc.

In my experience the vast majority of Lab Directors follow the above ethical codes to the letter. I have only seen a few instances of a Lab Director deviating from what I though was acceptable ethical conduct. The first story involves the same pharmacist-businessman and Regional Reference Lab as referenced in the chapter above. The Regional Reference Lab had a small satellite lab in the small town where I lived. It was mainly a draw station with most of the testing being sent to the big city where that lab had its headquarters.

The businessman-pharmacist and the Regional Reference Lab were competitors. From the start they did not get along, and their relationship would further sour over time.

A few years after setting up the main lab described in the prior chapter the pharmacist-businessman asked me to take on the Lab Directorship for a mid-size outpatient clinic. The clinic was doing a few moderate complexity tests on point of care testing equipment, so they needed a Pathologist to be Lab Director. I said yes I could take on that position; it would not be a conflict of interest with any of the other positions I held.

I knew before taking on the Lab Director position that lab had formerly done business with the Regional Reference Lab. I assumed that there was nothing wrong with the switch of that clinic from one lab to another.

About a month later, one of the Lab Directors from the Regional Reference Lab called me. This Lab Director made an allegation that the pharmacist-businessman had gotten the clinic to switch labs based on offering lower prices for testing. I said there is nothing wrong with that. America is a capitalist country; that is perfectly legal.

The Regional Reference Lab Director made allegations that there had been an improper inducement for the clinic to switch to the pharmacist-businessman's lab. I said that I was not party to the negotiations between the clinic and the pharmacist-businessman. I am just an employee and do not have ownership interest in the business; thus I do not sit in the closed door meetings. I said I'd ask the pharmacist-businessman if there had been any improprieties.

The Regional Reference Lab Director said that the the transaction amounted to "bribery" and threatened legal action. I said that the statutory definition of bribery is an improper inducement to a government official to influence the government official in the discharge of his or her duty. Neither the clinic owners nor the pharmacist-businessman are government officials, nor do they conduct business directly with the government. Hence this cannot be bribery.

The Regional Reference Lab Director then threatened to sue alleging breach of contract. He alleged that an improper inducement had caused the clinic to break its contract with the Regional Reference Lab.

I said that my lawyer is Mr.____. You can serve the lawsuit papers on my lawyer. Be advised that if you sue me, I will counter-sue you alleging harassment and monopolistic business practices. If you lose the lawsuit you will have to pay me for wasting my time. I will charge you something punitive, like $500 per hour, for wasting my time.

The phone call ended at this point and I immediately called the pharmacist-businessman, followed by a phone call to my private attorney. The pharmacist-businessman denied wrongdoing and claimed that there was no improper inducement.

My attorney called the pharmacist-businessman's attorney. The pharmacist-businessman's attorney had been party to the negotiations, and said there was no inappropriate inducement. I took this at face value. Contrary to popular opinion, in my experience one lawyer will not lie to another lawyer. Instead, they refuse to answer the question if giving a true answer would be against their best interests. I later talked to the clinic owners, and they also said there was no improper inducement.

My attorney told me that I was right, and the Lab Director from the Regional Reference Lab could get in deep trouble for making such a phone call. The phone call could be construed as harassment and/or intimidation. However, without any way to document the contents of the call, it would be my word against his word. The Regional Reference Lab should have had its lawyer contact the pharmacist-businessman's lawyer. The call should not have been made from Lab Director to Lab Director.

My private attorney sent a letter to the Regional Reference Lab attorney complaining about the Lab Director's phone call and instructing the Regional Reference Lab not to call me anymore. The letter further instructed the Regional Reference Lab to send all correspondence to my attorney and/or the pharmacist-businessman's attorney. I did not hear further from the Regional Reference Lab. They did not take any legal action that I am aware of (i.e. they were bluffing).

My attorney wanted to send a letter directly to the Lab Director of the Regional Reference Lab. This letter would inform the Lab Director that his actions were dishonest, unethical and probably also illegal. This proposed letter would warn the Lab Director against slander and liable. Slander and liable are defined as making false statements with the intent of causing damage. I told my lawyer not to send a letter directly to the Lab Director. The letter to the Regional Reference Lab attorney is sufficient. The Regional Reference Lab can handle the matter internally.

The take home points here are:

1. Always know as much as possible about a job position before taking it. In this case, I knew almost nothing about the clinic Lab Director position when I took it.
2. Let the lawyers do the lawyer work. Do not overstep the bounds of your office or perform work in areas where you have no expertise.
3. Lab can be a cutthroat business, just like any other business.
4. When two competitors go to war, try to stay out of the fight to the extent you can.
5. Always do the right thing. If you know you're in the right, you cannot be intimidated by threats of legal action.
6. Some of the basic principles of ethics include "Do not say or do anything to another person that you wouldn't want said or done to you", "Do not say or do anything that you would not want to

be public knowledge". The Regional Reference Lab Director said things to me that he probably wouldn't want anyone else saying to him.

The following story relates to the sale of a laboratory that occurred in 1995 in a municipality that I would later live in. I was not living in that municipality at the time and this entire story is composed of second and third hand accounts. Rumor and hearsay are defined as circulating stories that cannot be substantiated.

Sometime in the 1970s a businessman-Lab Director founded his own lab in a small municipality in the middle of nowhere. In 1995 he sold this lab to the same Regional Reference Lab discussed above. The sale price was reportedly $3,500,000. The terms of the sale were that the Regional Reference Lab gets all the equipment on-site, and the businessman-Lab Director gets to stay on as Lab Director of that lab after the sale. The Regional Reference Lab thinks that they were buying all of the equipment on-site at that lab.

After the sale is completed, the Regional Reference Lab found out that some of the equipment on-site was leased. In other words, the businessman-Lab Director did not own some of this equipment and could not sell it. The amount that the Regional Reference Lab overpaid was about $1,500,000 out of the $3,500,000 purchase price.

My assessment so far: There is a Latin saying "caveat emptor". It translates as "let the buyer beware". It is used as a legal term to imply that the buyer has the legal obligation to do due diligence, and properly investigate the situation before entering into the purchase. If this story so far is true, it means that the Regional Reference Lab did not do its due diligence before entering into the purchase agreement. Equipment leases are usual and customary in the Lab business, and the Regional Reference Lab should have done its homework better before going ahead with this purchase.

Supposedly, at this stage of the game, the Regional Reference Lab demands the return of $1,500,000 from the businessman-Lab Director. The businessman-Lab Director refuses. The Regional Reference lab retains an attorney that sends letters to the businessman-Lab Director threatening a lawsuit if the disputed monies are not returned. The businessman-Lab Director then tells the Regional Reference Lab that if they sue the businessman-Lab Director, he will quit as Lab Director of that lab.

My assessment so far: This is not unreasonable. It would not make sense to keep working for a company that is suing you.

The threat of the Lab Director quitting sends the Regional Reference Lab scrambling to find another Lab Director for that lab. The position requires someone on-site, it can't be done remotely. No other Pathologist lives anywhere near that small municipality. Lab Directors are extremely hard to find, especially for such a remote municipality.

The head of the Regional Reference Lab called in his subordinate Pathologists one-by-one and asked if they would voluntarily move to this remote municipality for a while until this is sorted out. They all refused. The head of the Regional Reference Lab then called in the lower ranking Pathologists and told them that he might send one of them to this remote municipality involuntarily. They all said that they would quit their jobs rather than move to this small municipality.

At this point, the Regional Reference Lab knows that it is caught in the proverbial "deal with the devil". The term "deal with the devil" is used metaphorically to describe a deal from which one would like to extricate oneself, but is unable to do so.

The Regional Reference Lab has to keep doing business with the businessman-Lab Director. If he quits as Lab Director at the lab in question, there would be no replacement. The Lab Director position would go vacant. Any lab without a Lab Director would be quickly shut down by the regulators, in this case, CMS. If this lab got shut down by the regulators, the Regional Reference Lab would lose the entire amount of money it put into the purchase. Supposedly, the matter is later settled with the businessman-Lab Director agreeing to pay back a much smaller amount than the $1,500,000 disputed amount.

As mentioned at the start of this story, it is entirely composed of unsubstantiated rumor and hearsay. Let's think about my ethics in repeating such a story. The story is educational and entertaining (beneficence). I haven't mentioned any of the parties by name, so there is no real damage done (non-maleficence). I can tell my stories to anybody I want (autonomy). I am willing to tell my stories equally to everybody in the whole world (fair and just distribution).

In a situation where you have not substantiated a story, do not repeat the story and/or do not repeat the names of the parties involved. If you repeat the names of the parties involved in the story you will make enemies of all the parties involved and you could get sued for slander and/or liable.

Chapter 28 – How to prevent lab mutinies

There is a saying that rich and powerful people are judged by how they treat the people below them. As a Lab Director you will be the most powerful person in Lab and also likely the wealthiest. In many ways, you will be judged by how you interact with the rank and file employees in Lab.

This story involves the large university hospital where I trained. I will call this "Hospital A" for the purposes of this story. The Lab Director for Hospital A had been present at the founding of the hospital in 1957. He set up the Pathology Department as a group which he owned. This was a brilliant move, and played in his favor for decades to come. I will refer to his pathology group as "Slavedriver Pathology Group" for the purposes of this story.

When I started training in 1991 at Hospital A the group had 7 Pathologists. The Lab Director was a very elderly gentleman by then in his early 80s. He was doing very little work, and delegating almost everything to the younger pathologists. He had been encouraged to retire, but refused to do so. He could not be forced to retire since he owned the group.

He had a reputation as a "slavedriver" assigning as much work as possible to the other 6 Pathologists in the group. They were his direct employees and he could force them to work as hard as possible. Since he owned the group, he stood to profit from this. The money that was not paid in salary added to his profit. Exploitation is defined as forcing people to work as hard as possible for as little pay imaginable.

This Lab Director also overworked the histotechs, secretaries and all other positions under his control. The way he did this was by intentionally leaving positions vacant. This lab had allotted slots for 11 pathologists but the slavedriver Lab Director did not want to do any hiring. Instead he wanted to make the existing Pathologists work harder. He did the same with all other job positions under his control. The result was poor morale and high turnover of essentially all positions in this lab.

Sometime in 1993 Hospital A acquired another hospital which I will call "Hospital B" for the purposes of this story. Hospital B is a nearby mid-size to large hospital with 4 pathologists. The plan was that the Pathology Departments for the two hospitals would be merged. The Lab Director of Hospital A wanted to lay off 2 of the 4 Hospital B Pathologists and centralize the Pathology services at Hospital A.

All the other pathologists objected to layoffs. The other Hospital A pathologists are already working like slaves, and the added work from Hospital B would send their workload into the stratosphere. The Hospital B pathologists object because they don't want to get laid off. The slavedriver Lab Director dug in his heels. He is going to lay off 2 of the Hospital B pathologists, and tells the other Pathologists they will have to tow the line because they are all just employees. This resulted in a series of arguments between the slavedriver Lab Director and the other pathologists. These arguments progressively worsened over time as the merger date approached.

About this time, the 6 Hospital A employee pathologists and the 4 Hospital B pathologists began having closed door meetings. The slavedriver Lab Director was not invited to these meetings. His absence from meetings was unusual since he headed the department. I did not sit on those closed door meetings. Later I found out that the pathologists were meeting to plan the ouster of the slavedriver Lab Director and form their own pathology group.

The 6 employee Pathologists from Hospital A and the 4 Pathologists from Hospital B approached the Hospital Administration of both hospitals. Both hospitals administrations and all pathologists met in one big meeting. The Pathologists threatened to resign en-mass. All ten will quit if there is any attempt to lay off any Pathologist, and force the other Pathologists to take monstrous workloads. The slavedriver Lab Director is called into this meeting. He again digs in his heels. He will lay off some Pathologists and make the others work harder. He figures that since he owns the group, he is untouchable. He is wrong.

Both hospital administrations involved know that their entire Pathology Departments are getting ready to resign en-mass. They cannot allow this to happen. If events play out this way their hospitals will be seriously damaged. The administrations of both hospitals help to unseat the slavedriver Lab Director.

The mechanics of his unseating are as follows. The 6 employee Pathologists from Hospital A and all 4 Pathologists from Hospital B form their own group. For the purposes of this story I will call this "Mutiny Pathology Group". Needless to say, the slavedriver Lab Director is not invited to join Mutiny Pathology Group. Both Hospital A and Hospital B revoke their contracts with Slavedriver Pathology Group and hire Mutiny Pathology Group on the same day.

Two weeks later, the slavedriver Lab Director shuffles off into retirement. Everyone in the department is glad to see him go. Not one person misses him.

I was not involved in the mutiny at Hospital A, and kept my distance from the proceedings. I was a pathology resident at the time. The trainees were seen as very low ranking and expected to be seen but not heard. The pathology residents had no say in the events that played out.

The Lab Director for Hospital A was a slavedriver for the pathology residents. The other residents and I did essentially 100% gross exams, working from 7AM to 9PM, working like we really were slaves, until this Lab Director was forced out. The other pathology residents all hated this Lab Director. I figured that the heavy workload was a rite of passage, similar to a "hazing" at a college fraternity. All these years later, I have no ill will to the slavedriver Lab Director, and figured that I learned a huge amount about gross exams working those long hours in his lab.

This sequence of events whereby rank and file employees unite to throw off a cruel boss very closely resembles the Mutiny on the Bounty. The Mutiny on the Bounty really did happen. It took place in the year 1789. I have seen at least three similar mutinies in my 23 year career, the most spectacular of which is given above. The other two mutinies involved administrative removal of lab supervisory personnel that were universally disliked by their subordinates.

The three lab mutinies I have seen occurred in different labs years apart from each other and thousands of miles away from each other. In each instance, I was not Lab Director, but instead in the Pathologist position or Pathology Resident position. In each instance, my job position did not require me to take any administrative action, and I kept my distance form the proceeding. Do not get involved in this type of situation unless you are required to. In my experience the pathway to mutiny involves:

1. An authoritarian supervisor with an attitude of "I am the boss". Typically a perfectionist with an expectation that everything should be done his or her way.
2. Seasoned rank and file employees that are not going to put up with the supervisor. The employees are good at what they do and they know it. They resent the dominating supervisor.
3. Slow buildup of resentment. The relationship between the supervisor and the employees deteriorates over time. The lab techs may begin to act passive aggressive, intentionally making mistakes to upset the supervisor. The supervisor being authoritarian, responds the only way he or she knows how – by repeatedly chewing out the lab techs.
4. The situation deteriorates further and faster. The lab techs increasingly feel that the supervisor is unapproachable and/or they don't want to have anything to do with the supervisor. The supervisor acts increasingly authoritarian as control slips away. The lab techs and supervisor will typically start reciprocal write-ups on each other at this stage if they haven't already done so.
5. The triggering event. In the story above it was the proposed layoffs. In the second mutiny I have seen, the supervisor asked the employees to pay out of pocket for tickets to a fundraiser dinner for a charitable organization that the supervisor headed. In the third mutiny I have seen, the triggering event was the supervisor withheld annual increments for a number of employees.
6. Open rebellion. The lab techs refuse to take orders from the supervisor and typically threaten a mass walk-out. At this stage, there are loud arguments in public areas. The parties involved have come to hate each other and will not conceal their hatred of the other party. There is likely going to be a huge number of write-ups between the parties involved.

As noted above, the triggering event can be very petty, but is causes the situation to explode. If you see a Lab Supervisor going down the pathway leading to mutiny, you must try to stop this at the earliest stage possible. In my experience, the further a lab goes down the pathway to mutiny, the harder it is to pull back from the brink and the more likely it is to run to completion.

You will be doing negotiation between the Lab Supervisor and the rank and file employees. You will be the go-between for the Lab Supervisor and the lab techs who feel that they cannot communicate with the Lab Supervisor. Meet privately with the Lab Supervisor and meet privately with the lab techs to discuss the situation. What do they want from each other? What can you offer to either party?

Try to defuse the situation to the extent you can. Bring all parties into one big meeting, and try to make peace. Offer whatever appeasements you can without offending any of the parties at the table. Be as diplomatic as possible. In this meeting, try to concentrate on points in common and do not dwell on the differences between the Lab Supervisor and the lab techs. It will take more than one meeting to patch up the differences. Hopefully, this first meeting can prevent things from getting worse.

It is imperative that you should be impartial. Do not take sides. You are an authority figure, much the same was that the Lab Supervisor is an authority figure; however, you must resist the temptation to join the battle on the side of the Lab Supervisor. Likewise, do not join the battle on the side of the lab techs.

I have seen a few instances where a series of meetings between the Lab Supervisor and lab techs probably prevented a mutiny. In the other cases, the mutiny ran to completion. Much of the problem relates to the personalities involved. You cannot change other people's personalities. If the Lab Supervisor is going down the pathway to mutiny, you must try to reshuffle the Lab Supervisor into a different position. Usually you can switch that person into a section supervisor position, and switch one of the section supervisors into the Lab Supervisor position.

I have never had a Lab under my command go into a full scale mutiny. If it happened, I would be on the phone to the Hospital Administrator telling the Administrator that the Lab Supervisor has to be removed immediately or the lab is going to stop functioning.

I have told these stories to many people and most do not believe they really count as mutinies. The definition of a mutiny is that it is an agreement among multiple individuals to stop following authority. There is no requirement that the action has to take place aboard a ship, and no requirement that the mutineers have to be military. Thus the stories given above really are mutinies whereby multiple Pathologists agree to stop following orders from the slavedriver Lab Director and multiple lab techs agree to stop following orders from their despised Lab Supervisor.

The point of these stories is that you always have to be nice to your subordinates. You cannot take their place in doing their work. You need them more than they need you. Never criticize unless absolutely necessary. Even then, phrase it in a constructive manner. Be quick to thank employees for a job well done. Try to find something that the lab staff excel at, and give them awards at least twice a year. Give awards for all goals met. Be sincere in your praise when handing out the awards.

You should motivate the people below you in a positive manner. Ask for the lab staff's input and opinions. Take seriously any suggestions for improving the lab. Do not overwork your employees unless absolutely necessary, and even then be generous with the overtime and thankful for their work. Be generous to the rank and file employees. Buy them lunches and dinners. Don't say or do anything to another person that you wouldn't want said or done to you.

Chapter 29 – How to chair a meeting

According to most hospital's bylaws, the Lab Directorship comes with automatic membership on some hospital committees and also typically comes with automatic chairmanship of the lab departmental meetings and automatic chairmanship of the Tissue and Transfusion Committee.

Blood utilization review is mandated by TJC and all hospitals will have such a committee. In my experience it is most commonly called the Tissue and Transfusion (T&T) Committee, but I have also seen it called the Blood Utilization and Transfusion Review (BUTR) committee. In almost all hospitals, the Lab Director chairs this committee.

Before I started my first Lab Directorship, I had been the member of several hospital committees, but had never been the chair. At the time, I was overloaded with slides to look at, and my committee membership was quite slack. I would pick a seat toward the back or behind someone else, so as not to be clearly visible to the people at the head of the table. I only spoke when asked to, completed all assignments in a timely manner, but never volunteered for additional work.

When I was promoted to Lab Director, the table was turned, in a literal as well as a figurative sense. I was assigned the chairmanship of two committees, and went from hiding at the back of these committees to sitting in the driver's seat. I quickly learned how to chair a meeting.

Your committee chair work will be assisted by a secretary, typically a secretary from the Medical Staff Office. The secretary will reserve meeting room space for the date and time of the meeting.

The work of chairing a committee begins well in advance of the meeting. You should prepare the agenda at least one week in advance of the meeting. The secretary will then E-mail the agenda to all members of the committee along with a reminder of the time, date and place of the meeting. An additional reminder E-mail should be sent to all committee members about 24 hours before the meeting.

The day of the meeting you should arrive early. Lead by example. The secretary will lay out multiple copies of the agenda, last month's meeting minutes and an attendance sign-in sheet in the meeting room. The secretary will take notes for this meeting and later type the minutes. Breakfast may or may not be served.

As people come in, remind them to sign the attendance sheet. This is important, since you need to document a quorum. Also, the physicians present typically have meeting attendance requirements needed for renewal of privileges every 2 years. If anyone comes but forgets to sign in, it counts as an absence for attendance purposes.

Count the number of members present, and call the meeting to order when you have reached a quorum. Typically a quorum is 50% plus one of the members. With the Tissue and Transfusion Committee, there was little attendance, and most months we didn't reach quorum. If quorum is not met, the session in the meeting room is called a "working session" instead of a meeting. You can still do most of the work of a committee, but anything requiring a vote has to be put off until there is a quorum.

Go down the agenda one item at a time. Start with the approval of last month's minutes. Looking over last month's minutes can jog your memory as to items that are important and need to be discussed again at the current meeting.

Most of the committee work will be unobjectionable. The statistics for blood usage will be presented. The blood utilization fall-out cases will be reviewed. For example Patient XYZ was transfused with a hemoglobin of 16 g/dL. This patient's chart has been pulled for the meeting. Review of the chart indicates a substantial gastrointestinal bleed. Everyone agrees that the transfusion is indicated. The case is closed.

If there is a case that is still seen as a fallout after chart review, it is referred to the department of the physician that ordered the transfusion. For example Patient Z got transfused with a hemoglobin of 12 g/dL and the indication on the chart and requisition form is "anemia". The physician that ordered the transfusion is a Family Practitioner so the case is referred to the Family Practice Department to review.

If the Family Practice Department feels the transfusion is indicted, the case is closed. If the Family Practice Department has a problem with the transfusion, they may mandate continuing medical education, or other remediation on the physician involved. The Family Practice Department may punt the case back to the Tissue and Transfusion Committee to do the investigation and remediation.

This is where the situation starts to get tricky. You will have a clinician coming into the Tissue and Transfusion Committee trying to explain why he or she ordered this particular transfusion. Usually, they will stick to their story - the patient was symptomatic, the patient needed oxygen carrying capacity, etc. I have only rarely seen a patient in person since finishing medical school 23 years ago and I was not present during that patient's physical exam, so I have no way of knowing if this physician is telling the truth or not. In this circumstance, you have to give the benefit of the doubt. The committee determines that the transfusion was indicated and the case is closed.

Even before the meeting starts I know that the case will likely be closed in that clinician's favor, just like virtually every other case in the history of the committee. While the clinician is there for the committee meeting I make sure the clinician is very clear on the indications for red blood cell transfusion. This is presented as an educational "oh, by the way, did you hear about our committee's transfusion criteria" and not presented as a corrective action.

While I have this clinician as a captive audience in my committee meeting, I am going to remind him or her of all the criteria for red blood cell transfusion at that hospital - bleeding with hypotension, bleeding more than 750ml or more than 15% of the patient's blood volume, hemoglobin less than 8 g/dL with symptoms of anemia, hemoglobin less than 10 g/dL in a preoperative patient, etc. In my experience, the combination of calling that clinician in front of a committee and informing that clinician of the transfusion criteria at that hospital almost always prevents recurrence of inappropriate transfusion.

The committee then moves on to other business, routine matters such as presenting statistics and approving the biannual renewal of the contract with the regional Blood Bank. Award letters are passed around for signatures thanking the champion blood donors who just completed their 30th, 40th, 50th donations, etc.

After finishing all the business, make a double check of the agenda to see that all items on the agenda were brought up at the meeting. Ask the members if there is any business that is not on the agenda but needs to be brought up. If there is no further business the meeting is adjourned with an announcement that the next meeting will be held the same day next month.

Immediately after the meeting is over, look at the attendance sheet and make a note of the absent physicians. Towards the close of the same working day, call these physicians one-by-one, informing them of the events that transpired at the meeting and reminding them that there is a meeting attendance requirement. Most will tell you that they were too busy to come, had a conflicting clinic schedule, etc. If any clinicians have not met 50% attendance over the past several months, ask them if they could send proxies, or turn their committee seats over to other physicians.

In my experience, the main job of the chairman is to keep the meeting flowing smoothly, and prevent the meeting from getting bogged down in one or more unimportant details. You don't need to be an expert in parliamentary rules of debate.

I bought a copy of Robert's Rules of Order, and found that at most meetings it was of little help. Even though there are few meetings where you will need a copy of Robert's Rules, make sure to keep a copy with you at all meetings. As detailed below, the need could come up at any time.

As the committee chair you are tasked with handling all procedural issues that come up in the meeting. If a procedural matter came up, and you didn't have a copy of Robert's Rules with you, you might not know how to proceed. In this situation you should table (i.e. postpone) that one item to the next meeting and research how to handle the procedural issue. Avoid making up the rules as you go along.

The most important point is that you have to be fair and impartial. If there is debate, allow both sides of the debate equal time. Make it clear to everyone that each side is allowed the same amount of time to present their case. That is more important than knowing all the intricacies of the parliamentary rules of debate.

In every meeting there is likely to be one or more person that likes to talk too much and/or likes to be the center of attention. If one person is talking for more than 5 minutes and not allowing anyone else to speak, interject as politely as possible that debate for this topic will be limited to another 2 minutes in order to discuss all topics at this meeting. Let the person talk another 2 minutes then politely but firmly tell him or her the meeting has to go on to other topics in order for the meeting to accomplish its agenda in the time allotted.

Not many issues needed to be voted on, and few of these issues were contentious. There were only a few instances where the debate seemed to trail on and on. When this happens, interject that you are setting a limit of 10 minutes for the debate. After the 10 minutes are up, close the debate and bring the matter to a vote.

In my many years experience as a chairman, there was only one instance where a clinician was called into a meeting and became very defensive. This was a case of red blood cell transfusion fallout. Transfusion was given to a patient with a hemoglobin around 9.5 g/dL. The clinician must have known he did something wrong. Instead of trying to justifying the transfusion, he attempted all sorts of parliamentary maneuvers such as quorum call, points of order, question of privilege, motion to table discussion, etc.

Luckily, I had brought my copy of Robert's Rules with me. As each motion and point of order was made, I'd look in Robert's Rules to see how to handle it. This slowed the committee meeting to a snail-pace but the work did eventually get done. The committee determined that the case did not require a corrective action. The case was closed in the clinician's favor, in spite of the parliamentary maneuvering and in spite of the fact he never tried to justify the transfusion.

If the case had been of a serious nature, I would have called in the hospital Medical Director to take over chairmanship of that particular meeting. The hospital Medical Director chaired multiple committees that routinely dealt with physician discipline. Thus, the Medical Director was much more experienced with parliamentary maneuvering and much more proficient at dealing with it than I was. Always know your limits, and be prepared to call in an expert if necessary.

Chapter 30 – Lab Director hiring, orientation, competency testing and retirement

The CLIA requirements for a high complexity testing Lab Director are given in 42 CFR § 493.1443.

The requirements for a moderate complexity testing Lab Director are lower. However, in the typical hospital lab there is a mix of waived, moderate and high complexity testing. The Lab Director needs to meet the criteria a for high complexity testing Lab Director or the lab will be cited for doing testing that the Lab Director is not qualified to direct. Thus, the criteria given in 42 CFR § 493.1443 serve as the minimum hiring criteria for the Lab Director of the typical hospital lab.

There are several permutations that would meet CLIA requirments. The most common situation requires that the Lab Director must be an MD, DO, or DPM and must possess a current medical license issued by the State in which the laboratory is located, and must be certified in anatomic or clinical pathology, or both, by the American Board of Pathology or the American Osteopathic Board of Pathology. The other permutations involve qualifications that CLIA considers equivalent.

CLIA allows an MD, DO, or DPM that is not a Pathologist to be a high complexity testing Lab Director if the practitioner meets the following criteria: must possess a current medical license issued by the State in which the laboratory is located, must have at least one year of laboratory training during medical residency (for example, physicians certified either in hematology or hematology and medical oncology) or have at least 2 years of experience directing or supervising high complexity testing. In my experience, this is limited to Lab Directors of labs doing subspecialty hematology/oncology testing. I do not know of a general hospital Lab Director meeting these criteria.

CLIA allows the Lab Director to have an earned doctoral degree in a chemical, physical, biological, or clinical laboratory science if certified by a board approved by HHS. Although CLIA allows this, it is generally only done in subspecialty laboratories. For example, a person with a PhD in Microbiology and Board Certified by the American Board of Medical Microbiology could serve as Lab Director for a microbiology laboratory, but not for the typical hospital lab.

The Lab Director at a hospital lab also doubles as the Clinical Consultant. There typically isn't enough work to justify one person for each position so one person typically carries out the work of both positions. In all States, medical consultations require an MD, DO or possibly a DPM degree and medical licensure by the State.

Thus the combination of the CLIA requirements and the State's requirements for medical licensure preclude anyone other than an MD, DO or possibly a DPM from acting as as simultaneous Lab Director and Clinical Consultant at a hospital lab.

There are unusual permutations that would be acceptable under CLIA. For example separating the Lab Director and Clinical Consultant positions, allowing someone with an earned doctoral degree in science and certified by a board to serve as Lab Director. The Clinical Consultant duties could then be delegated to any physician licensed in the same State as the Laboratory.

This permutation was attempted at the hospital mentioned above that could not find a Lab Director for more than a year. It was basically a desperation maneuver; the CMS was threatening regulatory closure if that hospital did not find a Lab Director immediately. The CMS allowed this permutation of PhD Lab Director plus MD Clinical Consultant temporarily on the understanding that the hospital was making a good faith effort to hire an MD or DO board certified Pathologist into the Lab Director position.

In my 23 years experience in Pathology and Lab Medicine, this is the only instance I know of where the Lab Director position was split from the Clinical Consultant position, with each position occupied by a different person. Since it was a desperation maneuver on the part of a lab facing regulatory closure, I assume this is not the normal state of affairs, even though it is allowed under the CLIA regulations.

In my experience Lab Directors tend to be older Pathologists that are cutting back on their work as they age. I am not much different than the average. When I graduated from training in 1996, I took a Pathologist position at a small municipal hospital. As the Lab Director of that hospital slowly aged and cut back on work I was assigned more and more of the Lab Director duties. He retired in 2005 at which time I was promoted to the Lab Director position vacated by his retirement.

Sometime around 2004 the pharmacist-businessman referenced in chapter 26 started his lab for which I was hired as Lab Director. By 2007 that lab had grown to be a large, full service outpatient lab.

Thus over the course of many years I went from being only a Pathologist to both Lab Director and Pathologist. In 2013 I would cut back on the Pathology, and end up predominantly to exclusively a Lab Director. This is the typical pathway to being a Lab Director, with the exception that I am retiring to Lab Director work a little early in life compared to most others.

In terms of recruitment, good luck. Lab Directors are harder to find than Pathologists, Pathologists are harder to find than lab techs, and a good lab tech is hard to find. If your lab is essential to its municipality, and having regulatory problems, give me a call. I might try my hand at fixing it up. Otherwise you will be placing advertisements on the internet and in pathology publications such as CAP Today, AJCP, Laboratory Medicine, etc.

When I took my current Lab Director position in a small municipal hospital lab, my orientation lasted maybe two weeks and occurred coincident with the preparation for a CMS inspection. Thus I was signing the manuals in preparation for a CMS inspection at the same time I was reading them for orientation. Reviewing the remainder of the lab's paperwork, such as QA manuals, competency evaluations, preventive maintenance logs, etc. took another three weeks. I have never seen another person start work as a Lab Director, so can't speak as to how long someone else might need for orientation.

Under CLIA the Lab Supervisor is charged with all competency evaluations in Lab. This includes the Lab Director position. This arrangement for the Lab Director's competency testing is problematic. The Lab Supervisor does not have an MD, but is being called upon to evaluate the work done by an MD. This evaluation is beyond the training and experience of a Lab Supervisor.

This arrangement also is conflicted, since the Lab Supervisor is subordinate to the Lab Director. The conflict of interest arises from the Lab Supervisor's temptation to write his or her immediate supervisor a good evaluation, and suppress any derogatory information.

In my 23 years in Pathology and Lab Medicine, I have only had one instance whereby the Lab Supervisor wrote a less than stellar evaluation of me as Lab Director. In the preceding CMS inspection, there were a number of problems in the chemistry section whereby the Lab Director position was cited along with the chemistry section. These types of citation on the Lab Director position are common, and do not reflect the job performance of the Lab Director per se but occur secondarily to a citation occurring elsewhere in Lab. The Lab Supervisor was new on the job, and carried the CMS citations onto my evaluation.

When I received this evaluation, I thanked the Lab Supervisor for taking the time to write the evaluation, and politely said that the CMS citations on the Lab Director position were unrelated to the job performance. I was as polite and tactful as possible.

Keep in mind that other people are entitled to their opinions. Their opinion of you may not be the same as your opinion of yourself; but still they are entitled to their opinion. It is very difficult to evaluate the job performance of an administrative position such as a Lab Director position. Hence, all evaluations are an opinion, and the Lab Supervisor is entitled to any opinion at all.

As Lab Director your job turns not on the Lab Supervisor's evaluations, but on the opinion of the medical staff at the hospital where you work. If the other doctors think highly of you, you will be able to stay in that job forever, well into old age. If the other doctors think poorly of you, your days on that job may be numbered.

As a Lab Director you are subject to Ongoing Professional Practice Evaluation (OPPE) at least every 6 months if you work in an institution accredited by TJC. You will be evaluated by your immediate supervisor the hospital Medical Director. The hospital Medical Director is likely to be of a different specialty, and have little knowledge of Pathology. Furthermore, you are in an administrative position, and evaluation for such positions is difficult.

In some instances the Medical Director has evaluated me based on meeting attendance, personality, appearance, absence of complaints, and overall lab turnaround time. In other instances, the hospital Medical Director did not know what to put down, and asked me what he should put down on my OPPE. In those circumstances, try to be modest while writing your own evaluation.

Lab Directors are also subject to Focused Professional Practice Evaluation (FPPE). Triggering events include your hiring to a new hospital, you apply for increased privileges, and/or you have made one or more mistakes significant enough to trigger an FPPE. I have changed jobs twice in my 23 year career in Pathology and Lab Medicine. Each move presumably triggered an FPPE. I never received a copy of any FPPE forms that resulted. Since Lab Director positions are administrative, it would be hard to imagine a need to increase privileges. I am not aware of any Lab Director ever receiving an FPPE due to performance issues.

I have seen numerous voluntary retirements of Lab Directors. In most instances the medical staff and administration was begging the retiree to stay, and felt that it would be impossible to find a replacement. I have only seen Lab Directors removed for cause six times:

1. Story #1 – major shift in INR. This happened in a small municipality about 125 miles from where I worked at the time. A lab tech receives a new lot of INR reagent and began using the reagent without recalibrating the analyzer or resetting the analyzer to use the ISI of the new lot. The tech continued using the controls from the old lot. The tech apparently did not realize that he was using a new lot of INR reagent. This resulted in a major shift in INR, the results were far too low. The shift persisted for weeks before it was discovered. In this time, one patient died of intracerebral bleeding and a dozen others had major bleeding episodes. The tech and Lab Director of that lab were fired.

2. Story #2 – Inappropriate relationship. A male Lab Director in his late-60s had an ongoing inappropriate relationship with a much younger female lab tech working in the same lab. The Lab Director and lab tech were married to other people, not married to each other. The Lab

Director and lab tech did not try to hide the relationship from the other people in Lab. The hospital administration found out and forced the Lab Director to retire.

3. Story #3 – Lab Director not in touch with the modern day world. The Lab Director in this story is around age 75. He has been working at the same hospital for over 40 years. He is living in the past and likes to talk about his glorious accomplishments in the 1960s. He hates computers, hates Ipads, doesn't like cellphones, and can't figure out most modern technology. More than 20 years ago, he allowed an AS400 computer into his lab. This computer is now outdated, but he has been refusing to allow a new computer system into lab. The hospital is getting a new computer system. The Hospital Administrator calls in the Lab Director and tells the Lab Director that the existing computer system in lab is hopelessly outdated. The hospital has paid millions to get a new computer system and Lab is part of the deal. Since the hospital has already paid millions, the computer will go into lab. The Lab Director digs in his heels and refuses to allow this computer system into lab. The Lab Director is forced to retire involuntarily and the new computer system goes into Lab.

4. Story #4 – Lab Director disability. This same story was referenced in the chapter above on Pathologist retirement. In this story an 86 year old Lab Director develops Parkinson's disease and becomes wheelchair-bound. He is forced to retire involuntarily.

5. Story #5 – Lab regulatory closure. This same story was referenced in the chapter on regulatory scrutiny syndrome. This unfortunate Lab Director headed up a small private lab that was caught sink testing. Sink testing involves disposing of patient specimens and turning out fraudulent test results. The Lab Director in question almost certainly must have known what was going on in his own lab. When the CMS found out about it, they performed a regulatory shutdown on his lab immediately on the spot. This Lab Director lost his business, and was banned for a time from re-entering the business. He tried to re-enter the business after the banning period ended, but no one would hire him. This was a heavy price to pay, but on the other hand his Lab had committed the greatest sin in the laboratory world.

6. Story #6 – Mutiny on the laboratory. This is the story referenced in the chapter on lab mutinies. This elderly Lab Director was unseated by his 10 employee Pathologists in a disagreement over workload and layoffs. This Lab Director was in his early 80s at the time, and retired after being forced out from his job.

Of these stories above #2, #5 and #6 were avoidable, #4 was unavoidable while #1 and #3 might have been avoidable. In any event, Lab Directors #1 to #4 would have had an appeals process spelled out in the hospital bylaws. Lab Director #5 would have had a CMS appeals process available. Lab Director #6 could sue for breach of contract.

Every hospital is obligated to follow its bylaws. In any ensuing lawsuit the plaintiff's attorney will look for ways in which the hospital did not follow its own bylaws. If the hospital deviates even one iota from its bylaws in a physician employee removal process, the physician employee will likely get reinstatement with back pay.

The Lab Director who became disabled would additionally have protections from the Americans with Disabilities Act (ADA) which requires a series of hearings before one can be removed from a job position. If the hospital deviates one iota from these requirements, the physician employee will likely get reinstated with back pay.

In my 23 years experience in Pathology and Lab Medicine I have changed jobs twice. The first time was related to salary, I took a higher paying job. The second time I moved was basically a retirement. I took a job with slightly less pay, but with much less workload.

Retiring from Pathology to Lab Director work is nice. I have plenty of spare time to do the things I like, such as writing this book. As mentioned above, I am up for any challenge involving fixing up a lab. If your lab is essential to its municipality, and having regulatory problems, give me a call. I might try my hand at fixing it up.

Made in the USA
San Bernardino, CA
16 March 2014

*there ain't no memories
in First Class*

With illustrations and original artwork
By Lowell Davis

There ain't no memories in First Class

By Lowell Davis

Red Oak II Books
Carthage, Missoura.

There ain't no memories in First Class

All Rights Reserved © 2005 by Lowell Davis

No part of this book may be reproduced or transmitted in any form or by any means, graphic, electronic, or mechanical, including photocopying, recording, taping or by any information storage or retrieval system, without the permission in writing from the publisher.

Published by Red Oak II Books

Printed in United States of America